SAFETY GUIDE

for Health Care Institutions

Fifth Edition

By Linda F. Chaff

 American Hospital Association

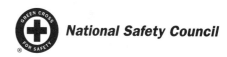 *National Safety Council*

AHA books are published by American Hospital Publishing, Inc., an American Hospital Association company

The views expressed in this publication are strictly those of the author and do not necessarily represent official positions of the American Hospital Association or the National Safety Council.

Library of Congress Cataloging-in-Publication Data

Chaff, Linda F.
    Safety guide for health care institutions / by Linda F. Chaff.—
5th ed.
      p.   cm.
    Includes bibliographical references.
    ISBN 1-55648-126-8 (pbk.)
    1. Hospitals—Safety measures.   2. Health facilities—Safety
measures. I. Title.
    RA969.5.C43   1994
    362.1'1'0684—dc20

                                      94-29435
                                         CIP

AHA Catalog no. 181149
NSC Product no. 12959-0000

©1994 by American Hospital Publishing, Inc.,
an American Hospital Association company

All rights reserved. The reproduction or use of this book in any form or in any information storage or retrieval system is forbidden without the express written permission of the publisher.

Printed in the USA

AHA is a service mark of the American Hospital Association used under license by American Hospital Publishing, Inc.

Text set in Souvenir Light
3M—10/94—0383

Audrey Kaufman, Acquisitions and Development Editor
Nancy Charpentier, Production Editor
Peggy DuMais, Production Coordinator
Susan Edge-Gumbel, Cover Designer
Marcia Bottoms, Books Division Assistant Director
Brian Schenk, Books Division Director

Contents

List of Figures and Tables

About the Author

Linda F. Chaff is a nationally respected safety expert who developed a strong safety foundation while director of protection services at Monongalia General Hospital in Morgantown, West Virginia. She also serves on many service-oriented committees and is a member of several national associations, including the National Safety Council and the American Society for Healthcare Risk Management. She is a member of the executive committee of the health care section of the National Safety Council, and has chaired state and national health care committees.

As president of Chaff & Co. Corporate Communications, Chattanooga, Tennessee, Linda publishes books and training manuals. She also develops and markets interactive training workshops, including *People Power,* a dynamic program that helps people perform more effectively by developing more positive attitudes. Her company provides consulting services for health care facilities on safety, health, and environmental issues. Linda also frequently authors published articles on safety, loss prevention, and training concepts and methods.

Safety Guide for Health Care Institutions is used extensively in health care facilities, colleges, and seminars both as a training resource and authoritative reference. Linda is the author of other publications including, "Managing Health Care Hazards," "Building a Successful Safety Committee," "Reporting Regulations for Hazardous Chemicals," and "Effective Health Care Facilities Management."

Linda has been awarded the Russell L. Colling Literary Award by the International Association of Hospital Security and Safety for a book she authored on health care security, *Safety Training Manual and Study Guide for Healthcare Security Officers.*

Preface

Health care facilities operate in a unique environment. No other business brings together such a diversity of services, people, and equipment. Unlike other services, providing medical care demands human performance with no margin for error, 365 days a year, 24 hours a day, with no downtime, holidays, or lapses in service.

Health care institutions are entrusted with the safety of several distinct groups—employees, visitors, volunteers, and, increasingly, members of the community—as well as the life and health of patients. In many cases, particularly in long-term care or psychiatric facilities, patients are unable to care for themselves or ensure their own safety. As a result, unsafe acts, equipment failures, and other dangerous conditions in these institutions may have especially serious— even tragic—consequences. This unique environment makes safety a high priority.

Compounding the risks inherent in the operation of health care organizations are rapid and dramatic shifts in society and technology. The past 10 years have seen numerous changes unprecedented in their effect on health care. For example, infectious diseases pose formidable dilemmas for both society and medical facilities. Health care institutions must care for these patients compassionately and safely while ensuring employee safety. Medical technology continues to grow at a rapid rate, giving the industry tools that can greatly enhance treatment. At the same time, however, these new tools introduce new risks that must be managed. Changing demographics influence health care as greater numbers of people become geriatric and require special care.

Additionally, regulations affecting health care continue to multiply. Medical institutions must fulfill the requirements of both government and voluntary agencies. To do this, health care facilities must keep abreast of changes in standards and set up processes to ensure that the standards are met. Failure to do this can result in both criminal and financial liability.

Clearly, a comprehensive safety program is required that involves the commitment and participation of staff facilitywide. The benefits of such a program are many: (1) Accidents can be reduced, along with workers' compensation claims and lost work time. (2) Citations and penalties from regulatory agencies can be avoided through compliance with regulations. (3) Compliance with these regulations will assist in gaining accreditation from the Joint Commission on Accreditation of Healthcare Organizations. (4) Liability for accidents and injuries that occur on facility premises will decrease as facilities are made safer places in which to work. (5) Medical staffs will be better prepared for emergencies (such as fire or other disaster), limiting the potential for damage to life, health, and property. By encouraging all staff members to participate, health care facilities can establish a feeling of teamwork that will boost employee morale and productivity.

These advantages represent just a few of the benefits that effective safety management can provide. This manual outlines a comprehensive program for achieving these goals. Chapter 1 provides guidelines for planning the safety program and describes the four preparatory steps: obtaining administration support, conducting the needs assessment, setting priorities, and developing policies and procedures. Chapter 2 provides essential information on regulatory and voluntary compliance agencies affecting health care. The various components of the overall safety program—the safety committee, departmental safety, patient safety, hazardous materials management, bloodborne pathogens, waste disposal, fire safety, emergency preparedness, and environment and workplace health—are described in chapters 3 through 11. Chapter 12 provides guidelines for implementing an incident reporting system, and chapter 13 is devoted to safety training. Chapter 14 focuses on the unique needs of mental health facilities. Chapter 15 suggests motivational and incentive programs that can be used to improve safety awareness and employee involvement in the overall safety program. Finally, the key to success of any safety program is ongoing evaluation. Chapter 16 provides the steps necessary for development of an evaluation process.

No health care organization can afford to operate without a strong safety program. This text provides the framework and resources on which a comprehensive safety program can be built and tailored to the facility's unique needs.

Acknowledgments

With considerable gratitude, I offer my thanks to everyone who contributed their time, knowledge, and skills to the revision of this book.

I am deeply grateful to Bob Britt whose technical and analytical skills were invaluable throughout the project. His commitment and perseverance, despite a hectic schedule, greatly contributed to the completion of the manuscript on time. In addition, I am indebted to Ann Marie Curtis whose technical writing and editing skills greatly assisted the completion process.

Joe McFaddin (safety director of Rose Medical Center), Mike Peltier (section administrator of the National Safety Council's Health Care Section), and Jodey Schonfeld (National Safety Council's technical publications manager) reviewed the manuscript for accuracy and provided critical comments and technical information during the whole procedure. I am thankful for their expertise and accessibility.

I applaud Audrey Kaufman, acquisitions and development editor, American Hospital Publishing, Inc., for her expertise in managing the publication of this book. Audrey was always available for guidance, especially around deadlines. Thanks, Audrey!

The following individuals actively participated in the revision by offering clear, concise information making the research process less tedious: Erik Auf der Heide, M.D., Gerald Baril, Leo Bosner, Dennis Bundy, Randy Burt, Frank Denny, Mellanie Ellexson, Steve Ennis, Albert Fala, Terry Fisk, Marshal Fowler, Linda Glasson, Sandy Griffin, Merrie Healy, Emma Hooks-Hébert, Eric Joseph, Matthew J. Key, Kristi Koenig, M.D., MaryAnn L. Northcote, Barbara Ondrisek, Tony Parente, Dan Peterson, Roger Pugh, Paul Russell, Robert Rusting, Ed Savard, Carl Shultz, M.D., Kenneth Smith, Ronnie Solomon, Emma Truett, Dave Wacker, Ron Wade, David Woodrum, Art Yow, and Pier-George Zanoni. I appreciate their effort in this endeavor.

The dedication and support of everyone involved at each stage of the project was outstanding and is thoroughly appreciated. Truly, the effort of so many people and their willingness to contribute made the revision of this book a delightful experience.

Safety Program Management

A health care facility is a complex institution comprising many diverse departments and functions. In addition to its primary responsibility of providing health care, it also must provide the services of a hotel, a restaurant, a retail business, a cleaning service, a laboratory, and so on. Because these services are so different, the departments that administer them tend to operate autonomously. Thus, each department within the health care facility generates a unique set of risks. The result is that within the overall facility a variety of risks often are managed in an uncoordinated, disjointed way.

Because of the tendency of departments to act independently of one another, and because of the complexity of routine facility operation, thorough planning and coordination are essential to a comprehensive and successful safety program. Within the health care institution, the process of establishing a successful safety program depends on (1) obtaining commitment from all sectors of the facility, particularly senior management; (2) conducting a facilitywide needs assessment; (3) identifying priorities and instituting preventive measures; and (4) developing safety guidelines in the form of written policies and procedures. These four preparatory steps are at the foundation of a results-oriented safety program.

In addition to dealing with internal considerations, health care facilities are faced with the major task of ensuring that their safety programs comply with a growing number of federal, state, and local regulations. Because compliance inspections by the Occupational Safety and Health Administration (OSHA), the Environmental Protection Agency (EPA), and the Joint Commission on Accreditation of Healthcare Organizations (JCAHO) often are unannounced, facilities must evaluate their safety programs aggressively and frequently.

This chapter provides guidance in the basic elements involved in setting up a successful safety program. These elements include:

- Gaining administration support
- Performing a needs assessment
- Setting priorities
- Developing policies and procedures
- Ensuring continuous safety performance improvement
- Changing the safety environment

☐ Gaining Administration Support

The most successful safety programs have one thing in common: All the facility's employees are motivated to work safely. This motivation comes not only from the individual employee's desire to avoid injury, but also from management's desire to demonstrate that safety and health are important aspects of every employee's job. Successful safety and health programs encourage employee participation, establish department head accountability, and visibly involve supervisors in the process.

The safety program should include a statement by top management that reflects the facility's mission and values. This statement provides the basis for the development of long-term safety goals and should be distributed to all staff members. It should include the following:

- A commitment from top management, including the board of trustees, to support and facilitate the safety program
- The contribution of the safety program to the goals of the facility
- The assertion that safety is a major element of department head and employee performance reviews
- Recognition that the safety objective is as important to the facility as its business objectives
- Goals for safety performance
- The goal to involve and empower employees to accept personal responsibility for their own safety
- The requirement to ensure ongoing performance improvement

☐ Performing a Needs Assessment

A *needs assessment* is a survey of the current programs, prevailing attitudes, and risks presently affecting facility operation. Once the needs assessment has been completed, areas for improvement can be identified and a comprehensive program incorporating time frames and priorities can be developed.

Preparing for the Needs Assessment

A health care facility can conduct a needs assessment in one of two ways. These are:

1. The facility can use outside resources (for example, consultants, teams from other facilities, and insurance company risk management/loss prevention staff).
2. The facility can use in-house resources.

The advantage to using an outside resource is that the needs assessment is performed by people who are familiar with federal, state, and local regulations and are knowledgeable about successful safety programs in place at other facilities. Additionally, assessments performed by outside resources tend to be more objective than those done by in-house resources. Some disadvantages to using outside resources include the lack of ownership of the assessment and the fact that the facility may not gain as broad an understanding of problems as it would if the survey were performed internally. However, these disadvantages can be overcome by having an internal team work with the outside resource.

If the assessment is to be performed using internal staff, the survey team should comprise the safety director and representatives from administration and supervision, as well as other employees. Individuals with expertise in safety, hazardous materials, or materials handling should be included as needed. To facilitate the process and to contribute their perspective of safety performance, department managers should join the team during inspection of their departments. The internal assessment process will help develop cooperative relationships and the teamwork essential to making changes to the existing safety program.

The survey team should be trained in the goals and objectives of the assessment and should agree on the approach to be used. It should survey employee perceptions of safety support and any elements of the safety program that might be deficient, such as training, information management, and incident follow-up. If a more comprehensive survey of the entire safety program is to be done, it should involve random sampling of all employees.

One useful tool for conducting the needs assessment is a checklist. Many good resources exist for developing checklists, including OSHA and the JCAHO. (See appendix C at the back of this book for a prototype.) Hazard surveillance checklists completed by the facility can also be reviewed.

A comprehensive needs assessment includes a review of all of the facility's pertinent records. The records that organizations keep can give the survey team a sense of the current safety program's direction, including past accomplishments and oversights. Records that should be reviewed include:

- Accident/incident reports
- Reports to the board
- Internal inspection reports
- Safety committee minutes
- JCAHO survey reports
- Government agency inspection results, including those from OSHA, the EPA, state and county health departments, and fire departments
- Insurance company inspection records
- Workers' compensation statistics
- Policies and procedures
- Employee training records
- Internal inspection records

As part of preparation for the assessment, these and other records from at least the past 12 months should be gathered and summarized by the safety director. This will save time that the entire team would otherwise have to take to review every incident report from the past year. The documents should include statistics and trends such as the percentage of back injuries, needle sticks, slips and falls, and workers' compensation claims. If these documents are not available, it will be apparent that the facility's information management system is not in place.

Conducting the Assessment

For an assessment to be complete, it should include five elements. These are:

- Condition of the physical facility
- Employee perception
- Safety programs in place
- Condition of equipment
- Employee training

Condition of the Physical Facility

The safety of the physical facility can be determined using resources such as JCAHO standards, OSHA regulations, National Fire Protection Association (NFPA) Life Safety and Health Care Facility codes, and a checklist. Following are examples of items that should be included on the physical facility checklist:

- Have storage practices created a fire hazard?
- Are exit lights functioning?
- Are ceiling tiles in place?
- Are fire extinguishers inspected and in place?
- Are stairwells used as storage areas?
- Do fire doors function properly?
- Are exits blocked?

It is important that survey team members talk to the people who are most familiar with each particular area of the facility.

Employee Perception

Employees at all levels know the problems that exist with their safety program and, in many cases, can suggest solutions to specific problems. Their suggestions will be valuable to the team as it prepares recommendations for corrective action. In addition to soliciting employee perceptions about specific problems, the assessment team should survey employees to learn their perceptions of the overall safety climate within the workplace.

The survey can be done by either interviewing employees or asking them to complete a written form. Whatever approach is used, employees should be guaranteed anonymity. Following is a list of suggested questions that can be included in the perception survey:

- Does the safety program deal with the investigation of accidents and incidents in a positive manner?
- Are supervisors involved in accident prevention?
- Is safety considered important, and is good safety performance recognized at all levels of the organization?
- Do managers and employees communicate freely on safety issues and meet to formulate behavior-oriented safety goals?
- Do employees receive comprehensive safety training?
- Are safety inspections regular and effective?
- Does the facility take a strong but fair approach to safety rule infractions?
- Is there an effective system for dealing with reported hazards?
- Is the workplace climate conducive to adopting safe habits and work attitudes?

Many other types of questions may be included in a perception survey, and each facility must carefully tailor the survey to its own needs. Once complete, the survey provides management with the information necessary to make changes in policies and procedures and with the justification that management needs to make changes in the safety environment.

Safety Programs in Place

In addition to surveying employee perception of safety in the workplace, the assessment team needs to evaluate the effectiveness of the safety programs already in place. To do this, the team needs to review records to determine the following:

- Does the safety committee meet regularly?
- Is it structured properly?
- Are there data-tracking records showing that safety problems are corrected in a timely manner?
- Are there written policies for all safety requirements?
- Are the safety policies recent and reviewed annually?
- Are there specific policies for individual departments as well as the overall facility?
- Are the written procedures understandable and effective?
- Is training up-to-date, and have skill tests been performed?
- Has the effectiveness of the training program been reviewed and action been taken to correct deficiencies?
- Are training materials recent and in compliance with regulatory and JCAHO accreditation requirements?
- Is there an effective program that treats and manages employee injuries?
- Is there a workers' compensation cost containment program in place?

Condition of Equipment

The survey team also should determine whether a system of preventive maintenance is in place. This can be done by reviewing selected maintenance records. The goal of this review is to determine the following:

- Is there an "alert" or recall program in operation for defective equipment?
- Is defective equipment repaired or discarded?
- Is broken equipment allowed to be used?

Employee Training

Employee training is a very important element in the needs assessment. Policies and procedures are of little value if employees do not receive or retain the information they need in order to work safely. The assessment team should choose a representative cross section of employees from each department and test their knowledge of key elements of facility and department safety programs. Testing should include talking with employees to determine their understanding of specific regulations, for example, the OSHA Right-to-Know Law and the Bloodborne Pathogens Standard. Examples of the knowledge that employees should possess include:

- Where material safety data sheets (MSDSs) are located
- What hazardous chemicals they use
- What tasks involve exposure to bloodborne pathogens
- What action they should take in the event of exposure to blood or body fluids

The amount of testing can be reduced if records can be found that clearly show that employees have been trained and tested recently. However, if records either cannot be found or are poorly maintained, the team must spend considerably more time assessing the extent of employee knowledge.

Applying the Assessment Results

As mentioned previously, the needs assessment provides an in-depth look at the existing safety conditions within the health care facility. The assessment results enable the facility to focus on immediate as well as short- and long-term projects designed to eliminate existing safety problems and to anticipate safety problems in the future. Written policies and procedures can be used to help direct efforts and achieve safety goals. In addition, the assessment can foster a new relationship among administrators, managers, and employees. Because of ongoing interaction between the assessment team and the departments, employees feel that they are included in the decision-making process. This interaction builds employee commitment to the safety program and fosters a team effort for problem solving.

☐ Setting Priorities

The information generated by the assessment will need to be summarized in an assessment report. The completed report should be submitted to administration, and a follow-up meeting should be held to review the findings and set broad priorities. The survey team should not be disbanded until final priorities are set and approved.

Setting priorities for safety performance improvement is similar to any other process. The severity, frequency, and effect on employees are key factors to be considered. The prioritized results serve as the basis for development of long- and short-term goals. Written goals will prove useful in measuring the safety program's success. Additionally, seeing achievable short-term goals on paper will contribute to the participants' feeling of accomplishment.

□ Developing Policies and Procedures

After priorities have been identified and goals set, the next step is to develop or revise the policies and procedures that address these goals. Policies form the heart of the safety program. They outline the facility's commitment to the program, define responsibilities, and provide details for the development of procedures. Procedures can serve as a primary resource for safety training. Figure 1-1 shows a sample policy and procedure format.

Policies and procedures are evidence of the facility's intention to provide a safe environment for employees and patients. Additionally, these documents can be useful in defending the facility in the event of litigation. Moreover, the JCAHO requires policies and procedures for accreditation, as do government agencies such as OSHA.

One of the responsibilities of the safety director and the safety committee is to write and revise policies and procedures. (The role of the safety committee is discussed at length in chapter 3.) Policies must be developed for each major safety element—for example, accident prevention and reporting, hazardous material waste management, fire prevention, and so on. In addition, specific procedures must be written for each policy. For example, a hazardous chemical waste policy will include procedures for collecting, storing, and disposing of each different type of hazardous chemical waste.

When writing policies and procedures, the following areas should be addressed:

- *Policy:* The policy and the reasons for it should be briefly explained, as should its place within the framework of the entire safety program.
- *Responsibility:* The individual(s) responsible for ensuring that the procedures are followed and carried out should be identified by title. For example, "The infection control nurse has primary responsibility for coordinating the bloodborne infectious disease protection program."
- *Procedures:* The specific tasks of each participant should be indicated. Procedures should be step-by-step instructions that could be used in training.

Once they have been developed, policies and procedures should be approved in writing by the chief executive officer (CEO) of the facility and the chief officer of the medical staff, and should be reviewed at least annually for effectiveness, employee reactions, regulatory developments, and changes in operations. Additionally, policies and procedures should be consolidated into a policy and procedure manual that also includes the program goals; the authorization for the formation of the safety committee; the names of the safety committee members, chairman, and authority; and the statement of administration support. This manual can then serve as the comprehensive resource for the safety program.

□ Ensuring Continuous Safety Performance Improvement

It is essential to continually improve safety performance through strengthening facility performance goals and indicators. Performance improvement can occur most effectively if it involves some type of program that requires ongoing incremental changes that bring about proactive improvement, rather than reacting to a crisis.

Some forms of performance improvement are already being used in health care facilities to analyze and deal with safety problems. For example, in response to growing concern about infectious disease transmission, one department used a team approach to tackle the problem of needle sticks. Using available data, team members analyzed their sticks in a statistical manner, determining the major causes of the sticks and developing solutions to reduce their occurrence.

Continuous performance improvement in all areas of safety can be accomplished by using this same type of team approach to analyze safety problems. Teams meet on a regular basis to brainstorm and identify safety problems that should be addressed in order to reduce the

Figure 1-1. Sample Policy and Procedure Format

Hazardous Waste

Policy:

In keeping with (name of facility)'s policy of providing protection for its patients, employees, visitors and community, a program has been developed by (department responsible) to identify which wastes are hazardous and to ensure compliance with environmental regulations.

A waste is any solid, liquid, or contained gaseous material that we no longer use and either recycle, throw away, or store until we have enough to treat or dispose of.

The Resource Conservation and Recovery Act of 1976 (RCRA) requires anyone who generates or transports hazardous waste, or who owns or operates a facility for treating, storing, or disposing of hazardous waste, to notify the U.S. Environmental Protection Agency of this activity.

As a result of doing business, we generate wastes that can cause serious problems if not handled and disposed of carefully. These wastes could pose a danger to human health and the environment. They are considered hazardous, and are currently regulated by federal and state public health and environmental safety laws.

There are two ways wastes may be identified as hazardous:

• If they appear on a RCRA list
• If they are identified through specific characteristics

Responsibility:

A hazardous waste program coordinator will be appointed. The program coordinator will be the (title of person responsible) and will have the primary responsibility for the following:

• Call or write EPA for a "notification of hazardous waste activity" form
• Coordinate a task force on hazardous waste
• Obtain a list of hazardous wastes or substances as issued by the EPA and the state hazardous waste management agencies
• Assist departments in determining the quantity of hazardous wastes generated
• Report to the administrator in a standardized format total kilograms and an itemized list of actual and potential hazardous wastes generated by the facility
• Prepare and maintain the hazardous waste transport manifests
• Direct the hazardous waste program activities (for example, recordkeeping procedures, storing, training, choosing a transporter, reducing amounts of waste generated, cooperating with inspection agencies, reporting of incidents)
• Coordinate the development of department-specific procedures for handling and disposing of wastes

Department managers will have the primary responsibility to:

• Inform their employees who are at risk when handling or exposed to hazardous wastes and take appropriate measures to ensure their protection
• Initiate job safety training, if hazardous waste is generated
• Determine if a less hazardous chemical can be substituted for the hazardous chemical currently being used
• Ensure an MSDS is available for every hazardous waste

Procedures:

Guidelines have been established in accordance with EPA Rules and Regulations to help the (name of facility) department managers provide a safe working environment for their employees who handle hazardous wastes. The following information must be followed in complying with our program:

Waste segregation

• Do not mix hazardous with nonhazardous waste
• Do not mix incompatible waste from different hazard classes
• Additional lab pack guidelines (if used):

_____

_____

_____

Reprinted, with permission, from *Managing Health Care Hazards*. Chattanooga, TN: Chaff & Co., 1993, pp. 2–10.

chance of injuries or incidents. Often the brainstorming technique exposes serious problems that have been overlooked or ignored. Once the team has focused on a specific problem, team members use their experience to determine the root cause of the problem and to identify solutions. In some cases, statistical analysis is necessary. The information gathered must be passed on to the safety committee, the safety director, administration, and the board so that agreed-upon solutions can be implemented.

Once the necessary changes in procedures or practices have been made, the team can set new performance goals. It is important that such teams have the necessary training, technical support, and financial resources to help analyze problems and to avoid making changes that would create new and unexpected problems.

□ Changing the Safety Environment

Many health care facilities are beginning to realize that their safety programs do not meet their needs and must be revitalized. This realization may result from poor safety performance or recognition that the current program does not meet new standards set by regulatory agencies such as the JCAHO, OSHA, or the EPA.

If a significant improvement in safety performance is to be achieved, it will be necessary to undertake an aggressive approach in order to bring about a major change in the way the overall facility views safety. The objective of the change should be to replace old habits that no longer work with new beliefs, values, and behaviors that do work. Often this approach is referred to as changing the culture of an organization. Businesses worldwide have changed their corporate cultures in order to improve competitiveness in service, quality, and productivity, as well as to improve safety.

A desirable safety environment is one in which people at all levels of the organization know that they are valued. Examples of contrasting attitudes of undesirable and desirable environments are provided in table 1-1.

Changing the environment requires a significant amount of effort by all levels of supervision. Because employees need to understand the logic behind the changes in safety performance, they must be involved in the process of bringing about those changes. They need to be told hard facts about how poor safety performance affects the facility's ability to provide sound patient care and how failure to make the necessary changes will affect them personally. Employees want to know what new requirements are expected of them and, most important,

Table 1-1. Examples of Contrasting Attitudes of Undesirable and Desirable Environments

Element	Undesirable Environment	Desirable Environment
Response to pressure for increased safety:	Paperwork compliance	Focus on understanding why
Culture:	Fault or blame	Learning to improve performance
After an accident, attention is on:	What happened	Why it happened
Commitment to:	Form	Results
Response to problems:	Excuses	Apologies and new promises
Attitude:	Defensive	Ability to admit mistakes
Employee interaction:	Closed	Supervisors and employees openly discuss problems

Reprinted, with permission, from Peterson, D. Establishing good "safety culture" helps mitigate workplace dangers. *Occupational Health and Safety,* July 1993, p. 22.

how they will be involved. They want to be empowered to effect change rather than simply be led through the process.

Once change has been initiated, it must be kept going. Promotion of the change must go beyond what has been done in the past. Meetings, memos, presentations, publications, and everyday give-and-take interaction must be used to talk up the new environment. Because employees constantly struggle to sort out which ideas and instructions to take seriously, top management's message about the facility's intentions regarding safety must be clear and un-equivocal. And management must continue to send clear messages to remind employees that change is under way.

Implementing change in the safety environment requires financial resources and long-term commitment. Implementation should not be initiated unless the commitment is made and the resources are budgeted. Employees will easily recognize a lip-service commitment and many will resist attempts to change old habits to which they have grown accustomed. Thus, to avoid false starts that can seriously harm the implementation process, an understanding of what the change will require must be in place. Training, resources, commitment, and budgeting are abso-lutely essential elements in any attempt to change the safety environment.

☐ Conclusion

Four major preparatory steps—obtaining administration support, performing a needs assess-ment, setting priorities, and developing policies and procedures—provide the foundation for a successful safety program within the health care facility. Once the foundation is in place, the process of continuous improvement allows for a proactive approach to safety, rather than rely-ing on crisis management. This approach encourages teamwork organized by supportive management. When all these elements are in place, the facility will be in a position to provide employees, patients, and visitors a safe and healthy place to work, recover, and visit.

Regulatory and Voluntary Compliance Agencies

Throughout this century, patient care has steadily and dramatically increased in effectiveness. Because of advanced technology and procedures, patients with critical injuries and other acute conditions are more likely to survive today than ever before. Nevertheless, the same high-tech atmosphere that saves lives also brings more risks to health care employees, the community, patients, and the environment. For example, modern miracles of technology may malfunction or create electrical and fire hazards. Wonder drugs can have serious side effects. Substances that make treatment easier or more successful, such as anesthesia gases and radioactive materials, may pose hazards to employees and the environment. The everyday operation of a health care facility may engender numerous risks through unsafe conditions, such as wet floors or blocked fire exits.

These sources of risk have resulted in increased regulation by agencies seeking to ensure that health care facilities maintain a safe environment. These agencies can be divided into two principal types—governmental (regulatory) and voluntary. This chapter describes examples of both types and provides guidelines that facilities can use in dealing with regulatory inspections.

☐ Governmental Compliance Agencies

Governmental compliance agencies are those organizations that the government—federal, state, or local—has endowed with the authority to establish regulations and enforce them. Many times, the rules these agencies promulgate have the force of law and violators may be subject to fines, citations, and/or criminal penalties.

Governmental compliance agencies publish information and operate offices that concerned individuals can call on for answers or assistance. Contact information for each agency mentioned in this chapter is provided in appendix A at the back of this book.

Occupational Safety and Health Administration

In 1970, Congress passed the Occupational Safety and Health Act, which created an agency called the Occupational Safety and Health Administration (OSHA). Located within the U.S. Department of Labor, OSHA established regulations requiring employers to ensure safe and healthful working conditions for employees in the workplace. OSHA summarized the responsibility of employers in its General Duty Clause, namely that employers must provide "employment and a place of employment which are free from recognized hazards that are causing or are likely to cause death or serious physical harm [to employees]."

On the basis of this foundation, OSHA moved on to write regulations on both general and more specific safety issues for various industries. Once these regulations were established, it became the task of all employers and employees to implement and comply with the regulations.

OSHA has issued numerous regulations that affect health care facilities, especially in the area of general safety. For example, OSHA rules cover lockout/tagout procedures for machinery and equipment, ethylene oxide (EtO) exposure, entry to confined spaces, the use of ladders and scaffolds, electrical safety, and the use of personal protective equipment. Other areas of OSHA regulation and guidance for health care facilities include the storage and transportation of compressed gas cylinders, the control of waste anesthetic gas, the handling of cytotoxic (antineoplastic) drugs, and the use of X-ray equipment. Moreover, the Joint Commission on Accreditation of Healthcare Organizations (JCAHO) often relies on basic OSHA safety regulations in developing its accreditation criteria.

To control exposure to hazardous chemicals, OSHA enacted the Hazard Communication Standard in 1983. Under the Right-to-Know Standard, as it came to be called, all employees must be informed about the hazards of the chemicals they work with and how to protect themselves against these hazards. The Hazard Communication Standard has a number of specific requirements for employers, including establishing a written program and training for employees.

Because of growing concern about transmission of human immunodeficiency and hepatitis B viruses, OSHA enacted another major standard in 1991, the Bloodborne Pathogen Standard (BBPS). The purpose of this standard is to limit occupational exposure to bloodborne pathogens and other potentially infectious materials. The standard contains a number of requirements that are similar to those found in the Hazard Communication Standard. It requires a written exposure control plan and employee training. It also mandates universal precautions (that is, treating all body fluids/materials as if infectious) and emphasizes engineering and work practice controls. (See chapter 7 for a discussion of the requirements of the BBPS.)

OSHA enforces its requirements through workplace inspections. These inspections may occur for the following reasons:

- Imminent dangers
- Catastrophes or fatal accidents
- Employee complaints
- Programmed inspections for high-hazard industries
- Follow-up inspections

Inspections are conducted to determine whether safety and health hazards are being overlooked by the employer and, when necessary, citations are issued and fines levied.

If the potential harm represents an immediate threat to the health or life of employees, OSHA will take immediate steps to ensure that the hazards are eliminated. Otherwise, it may issue a citation that will result in penalties or civil or criminal fines. According to OSHA, consideration is given to the appropriateness of the penalty, the severity of the violation, the size of the facility, the good faith of the employer, and the record of previous violations. (See figure 2-1 for a list of OSHA regional offices.)

Many OSHA standards and guidelines relate directly to health care facilities. Implementing OSHA requirements can greatly enhance safety and the smooth operation of the facility. Resources exist to help the facilities understand OSHA requirements.

In 26 states it is not federal OSHA but a state occupational safety and health administration that regulates workplace safety and health. Although these entities must establish standards that are at least as effective as federal ones, they may—and on occasion do—establish *more stringent* standards.

U.S. Environmental Protection Agency

The Environmental Protection Agency (EPA) exercises control over the release of harmful materials into the environment and, like OSHA, has written both regulations and guidance documents. These rules and recommendations classify substances as hazardous to human health and the environment, outline procedures for handling these materials, govern the operation of waste disposal sites, and establish a system for dealing with environmental accidents such as leaks or spills.

Figure 2-1. OSHA Regional Offices

Region	Geographical Area Covered	OSHA Regional Office
I	Connecticut,* Maine, Massachusetts, New Hampshire, Rhode Island, Vermont*	133 Portland Street 1st Floor Boston, MA 02114 Telephone: 617/565-7164
II	New Jersey, New York,* Puerto Rico*	201 Varick Street Room 670 New York, NY 10014 Telephone: 212/337-2325
III	Delaware, District of Columbia, Maryland,* Pennsylvania, Virginia,* West Virginia	Gateway Building, Suite 2100 3535 Market Street Philadelphia, PA 19104 Telephone: 212/596-1201
IV	Alabama, Florida, Georgia, Kentucky,* Mississippi, North Carolina,* South Carolina,* Tennessee*	1375 Peachtree Street, N.E. Suite 587 Atlanta, GA 30367 Telephone: 404/347-3573
V	Illinois, Indiana,* Michigan,* Minnesota,* Ohio, Wisconsin	230 South Dearborn Street Room 3244 Chicago, IL 60604 Telephone: 312/353-2220
VI	Arkansas, Louisiana, New Mexico,* Oklahoma, Texas	525 Griffin Street Room 602 Dallas, TX 75202 Telephone: 214/767-4731
VII	Iowa,* Kansas, Missouri, Nebraska	911 Walnut Street Room 406 Kansas City, MO 64106 Telephone: 816/426-5861
VIII	Colorado, Montana, North Dakota, South Dakota, Utah,* Wyoming*	Federal Building Room 1690 1999 Broadway Denver, CO 80202-5716 Telephone: 303/391-5858
IX	Arizona,* California,* Hawaii,* Nevada,* American Samoa, Guam, Trust Territories of the Pacific	71 Stevenson Street Suite 420 San Francisco, CA 94105 Telephone: 415/744-6670
X	Alaska,* Idaho,* Oregon,* Washington*	1111 Third Avenue Suite 715 Seattle, WA 98101-3212 Telephone: 206/553-5930

*These states and territories operate their own OSHA-approved job safety and health plans (Connecticut and New York plans cover public employees only). States with approved plans must have a standard that is identical to, or at least as effective as, the federal standard.

As patient care becomes more and more complex, health care facilities must frequently deal with hazardous chemicals during routine operation. Whereas OSHA's Hazard Communication Standard covers the use of these substances by employees in the performance of their jobs, EPA rules apply primarily to the effects of the materials on the environment.

To effect a comprehensive system of control for dangerous wastes, the EPA has published numerous rules and guidelines. Following are those that have the greatest effect on health care:

- *Clean Air Act:* In 1970, Congress passed this act to empower the EPA to set permissible levels for the emission of hazardous substances into the air. Additional amendments were passed in 1990. These amendments listed 189 air toxics to be regulated, required that emissions leading to acid rain be reduced, and mandated the phaseout of certain chlorofluorocarbons such as Freon that reduce the earth's ozone layer.
- *Clean Water Act:* In an effort to buttress the 1972 Federal Water Pollution Control Act, the Clean Water Act was passed in 1977. This act limits the discharge of hazardous substances into waterways. It also established the National Pollutant Discharge Elimination System (NPDES), which requires permits for the discharge of harmful materials into water. In 1987, this act was reauthorized by Congress.
- *Toxic Substances Control Act (TSCA) of 1976:* This legislation regulates the manufacture, distribution, and use of toxic chemicals. It requires manufacturers to notify the EPA when proposing new chemicals, and it provides for the regular assessment of existing hazardous chemicals.
- *Resource Conservation and Recovery Act (RCRA) of 1976:* This is the act of most interest to health care facilities and other waste generators. It establishes a system for the control of hazardous wastes from the time they are generated until their final disposal, from "cradle to grave." The act divides waste generators into categories based on the amount of waste generated; requires permits for certain generators, transporters, and disposal facilities; and sets up a system whereby wastes are tracked from generation to disposal. (See chapter 6 for a complete discussion of RCRA's health care facility requirements.)
- *Comprehensive Environmental Response, Compensation, and Liability Act (CERCLA) of 1980:* Called Superfund, this act allocates funding and direction for cleanup of contaminated waste sites. It also confers liability on all involved with the waste site, even if they did not directly cause the contamination. Under CERCLA, hospitals have had to help pay for cleanup of waste sites to which they have sent their wastes.
- *Superfund Amendments and Reauthorization Act (SARA) of 1986:* This act reauthorizes and strengthens CERCLA. In addition, Title III of SARA establishes requirements for response in the event of an environmental disaster. Title III gives some hospitals additional environmental responsibilities (see chapter 6).

Taken together, these EPA regulations and guidelines establish a broad base of responsibility for health care facilities (see figure 2-2). Although the EPA is a major source of regulatory control, it also can act as an excellent source of guidance and information. The EPA publishes informative guides to help facilities understand and comply with its regulations. (See figure 2-3 for a list of EPA regional offices.)

Centers for Disease Control and Prevention

The Centers for Disease Control and Prevention (CDC) safeguards the health of the American people by controlling and preventing disease. It conducts research and publishes results—most often in the *Morbidity and Mortality Weekly Report.* This periodical is an up-to-date and thorough reference for health care facilities that want to stay ahead of new guidelines and regulations on topics such as infection control, infectious waste, and worker protection from bloodborne infectious diseases such as AIDS and hepatitis B. Various agencies, such as the JCAHO, OSHA, and the EPA, rely on the research and guidelines of the CDC.

The CDC has a growing number of national centers and offices that allow it to carry out a fight against disease worldwide:

- The National Center for Chronic Disease Prevention and Health Promotion works to prevent death and disability from chronic diseases.
- The National Institute for Environmental Health works to prevent death and disability due to environmental factors.

Figure 2-2. Laws Empowering the EPA

Law	Allows EPA to:
Clean Air Act, 1970	Set permissible levels for hazardous and visible emissions into the air
Clean Water Act, 1977	Limit discharge of pollutants into waterways (reauthorized 1987); set up the NPDES*
Toxic Substances Control Act, 1976	Regulate manufacture, distribution, and use of toxic chemicals
Resource Conservation and Recovery Act, 1976	Establish system by which wastes are tracked from "cradle to grave"
Comprehensive Environmental Response, Compensation, and Liability Act, 1980 (also known as Superfund)	Set aside funds for cleanup of contaminated waste sites; fix liability for contaminated sites
Superfund Amendments and Reauthorization Act, 1986	Reauthorize CERCLA; establish system of response for environmental disasters

*NPDES = National Pollutant Discharge Elimination System

Figure 2-3. EPA Regional Offices

Region	U.S. EPA Regional Office	Region	U.S. EPA Regional Office
I	John F. Kennedy Federal Building, One Congress Street, Boston, MA 02203, Telephone: 617/565-3420, Hours: 8:00 A.M.–5:00 P.M. EST/EDT	VI	First Interstate Bank Tower at Fountain Place, 1445 Ross Avenue, 12th Floor, Suite 1200, Dallas, TX 75202-2733, Telephone: 214/655-6444, Hours: 8:00 A.M.–4:30 P.M. CST/CDT
II	Jacob K. Javitz Federal Building, 26 Federal Plaza, New York, NY 10278, Telephone: 212/264-2657, Hours: 8:00 A.M.–5:30 P.M. EST/EDT	VII	726 Minnesota Avenue, Kansas City, KS 66101, Telephone: 913/551-7000, Hours: 7:30 A.M.–5:00 P.M. CST/CDT
III	841 Chestnut Building, Philadelphia, PA 19107, Telephone: 215/597-9800, Hours: 8:00 A.M.–4:30 P.M. EST/EDT	VIII	999 18th Street, Suite 500, Denver, CO 80202-2405, Telephone: 303/293-1603, Hours: 8:00 A.M.–4:30 P.M. MST/MDT
IV	345 Courtland Street, N.E., Atlanta, GA 30365, Telephone: 404/347-4727, Hours: 7:00 A.M.–5:45 P.M. EST/EDT	IX	75 Hawthorne Street, San Francisco, CA 94105, Telephone: 415/744-1305, Hours: 8:00 A.M.–4:30 P.M. PST/PDT
V	77 West Jackson Boulevard, Chicago, IL 60604, Telephone: 312/353-2000, Hours: 8:00 A.M.–4:30 P.M. CST/CDT	X	1200 Sixth Avenue, Seattle, WA 98101, Telephone: 206/553-4973, Hours: 8:00 A.M.–4:30 P.M. PST/PDT

Note: The geographical areas covered for the EPA regional offices are the same as those of the OSHA regional offices presented in figure 2-1.

- The National Center for Health Statistics monitors the health of the American people.
- The National Center for Infectious Diseases carries out work to prevent infectious diseases.
- The National Center for Injury Prevention and Control is involved in the prevention of nonoccupational injuries from both unintentional and violent causes.
- The National Center for Prevention Services carries out work to prevent vaccine-preventable diseases, HIV, sexually transmitted diseases, tuberculosis, and diseases from other sources.
- The National Center for Occupational Safety and Health works to prevent workplace-related injuries and illnesses.
- The Epidemiology Program Office provides epidemiological, communication, and statistical support and trains experts in epidemiology.
- The International Health Program Office is involved in strengthening the capacity of other nations to reduce disease, disability, and death.
- The Public Health Practice Program Office works to improve the effectiveness of public health delivery systems in promoting health and preventing diseases.

U.S. Food and Drug Administration

The Food and Drug Administration (FDA) is charged with supervising the development, testing, and monitoring of food and drug products and medical equipment. The FDA requires health care facilities to take corrective action to protect the safety and well-being of patients whenever information on a hazardous product is brought to their attention. It is the facility's responsibility to obtain, evaluate, and act on all information concerning hazards of the equipment, food, and medication it uses.

Until the mid-1970s, the FDA had no well-defined control over medical devices. In 1976, the Medical Device Amendments to the Federal Food, Drug and Cosmetics Act was passed to ensure safety and effectiveness of medical devices, including diagnostic products. The amendments require manufacturers to register with the FDA and follow quality control procedures. Some products must have premarket approval by the FDA, whereas others must meet FDA performance standards.

In 1990, Congress passed the Safe Medical Devices Act. The key requirements of the act include the following:

- Health care facilities must report incidents that suggest a medical device caused or contributed to a death, serious injury, or illness.
- Manufacturers must conduct postmarket surveillance on devices that are permanent implants and whose failure may cause serious health problems or death. Manufacturers must establish methods for locating patients who depend on these devices. As distributors of such devices, health care facilities must make certain information available to manufacturers for this purpose.
- The FDA is authorized to order device product recalls, issue stop-use notices, and impose civil penalties on health professionals and facilities for failure to do so.

Although the FDA keeps track of the performance of drugs, biologicals, and medical devices on the basis of mandatory reporting from manufacturers and user facilities, the reporting by health care professionals is voluntary. In 1993, the FDA established a new program called MED-Watch, aimed at encouraging greater voluntary reporting by health professionals of serious adverse health events and product problems. Physicians, nurses, and others who care for patients are the first to know when a drug or medical device does not perform as expected. The sooner the problem can be reported to the FDA, the faster corrective action can be taken.

A good source of information is the *FDA Desk Guide for Adverse Event and Product Reporting*. The guide contains examples of events to report and sample forms and can be obtained by calling the FDA.

U.S. Nuclear Regulatory Commission

The Nuclear Regulatory Commission (NRC) oversees operation of nuclear power facilities and regulates the handling, use, and disposal of radioactive materials. Hospitals may use radiological substances in several areas of operation: nuclear medicine, radiology, clinical laboratories, and research laboratories. The types of materials used in hospitals usually result in low-level radioactive waste.

Radioactive waste is unlike infectious and hazardous waste in that its danger can only be completely removed by time. Over time, radioactive materials decay and become less hazardous. The rate of radioactive decay, called the half-life, can be very slow; some materials require thousands of years to become thoroughly harmless. Meanwhile, these substances emit dangerous radiation, which has been associated with cancers, birth defects, and other health problems.

As a result, these materials must be carefully handled during use and adequately contained for disposal. Hazardousness and half-lives vary widely among radiological materials, as do disposal techniques. Contaminated materials may in certain cases be incinerated, allowed to decay in storage, or disposed of through the sanitary sewer, depending on their type and the applicable regulations. The NRC has published regulations governing these practices in its *Standards for Protection Against Radiation.*

☐ Other State and Federal Regulations

Other government regulations that need to be adhered to include those set by individual states and federal regulations such as those included in the Americans with Disabilities Act.

State Regulations

Individual states have requirements for health care facilities on many of the same topics as federal agency regulations. However, the state requirements may be more rigorous or extensive than federal standards. These state rules usually are enforced through licensure or the periodic inspection and relicensure process. States may regulate practices in many areas, including the following:

- *Occupational safety and health:* Federal OSHA gives states the option of implementing their own workplace safety and health programs instead of adopting the federal program. State OSHA programs must be at least as stringent as the federal program.
- *Hazardous waste:* States may establish their own hazardous waste management agencies to assist in compliance with EPA rules and possibly expand on them.
- *Infectious waste:* Although this is rapidly changing, the greatest source of rule making for infectious waste is state agencies. Regulations usually are issued by the board of health or the state EPA, if there is one. In addition, local sewer districts may have rules for the disposal of hazardous or infectious materials through the sewer.
- *Workers' compensation:* A common denominator for all states is the existence of workers' compensation laws, which generally are enforced by the state's attorney general or an agency that handles similar matters. The penalties for failure to comply with these laws, as well as the actual compensation to injured employees, are cumulative and can cause financial hardship for any size facility. Effective accident prevention and comprehensive safety programs can minimize unreasonable workers' compensation costs.
- *Fire and health codes:* The state or local fire authority, normally the fire marshal's office, verifies that fire safety requirements are met using its own state codes and National Fire Protection Association (NFPA) codes. In addition, health or fire department officials, or the authority having jurisdiction, will verify compliance with required infection control techniques, sanitation practices, proper storage and disposal of hazardous materials, and training of staff in proper identification and control of hazardous substances.

Because state and local requirements on these and other subjects may differ from or expand on national standards, it is crucial that health care facilities know the regulations that may affect them. As with federal mandates, facilities should be aware that regional requirements may change as new information becomes available. Abiding by state and local rules can provide a strong foundation for compliance with federal and voluntary standards.

Americans with Disabilities Act

To help the disabled live independently and become economically self-sufficient, Congress passed the Americans with Disabilities Act (ADA) in July 1990. This act provides comprehensive civil rights protection for 43 million disabled people in the following areas:

- Employment (Title I)
- Public services and transportation (Title II)
- Public accommodations (Title III)
- Telecommunications (Title IV)
- Other provisions (Title V)

Five federal agencies are responsible for enforcing and regulating the ADA. These are:

- Department of Justice (public services and accommodations)
- Department of Transportation (transportation)
- Equal Employment Opportunity Commission (employment)
- Architectural and Transportation Barriers Compliance Board (architectural standards)
- Federal Communications Commission (telecommunications)

The ADA prohibits prospective employers from discriminating against the disabled. According to the act, a qualified individual with a disability is one who satisfies the requisite skill, experience, education, and other job requirements, and can perform the essential functions of the position with or without reasonable accommodation. The act also states that any business or industry hiring the disabled must make reasonable structural or other process changes to allow a disabled person to perform the essential job functions. The act further provides that these changes should not cause undue hardship or expense to the employer.

Under the ADA, job descriptions must reflect the actual physical and mental requirements needed to perform the job. If an applicant is denied employment because an employer determined that the individual cannot perform the job, the job description becomes a critical issue in case of legal action against the employer.

Developing job descriptions requires careful analysis of the physical and force requirements, repetitions, and postures necessary to do the job. This careful analysis should not be relegated solely to supervisors or managers. Employers should draw on the skills of rehabilitation professionals who are skilled in job function analysis.

It is essential that facilities have written policies and procedures compliant with ADA guidelines. This will help the facility protect the rights of the disabled and avoid unwanted legal action.

☐ Voluntary Compliance Agencies

Just as there have always been not-for-profit health care facilities that have, in a way, "volunteered" medical services to the community, a parallel trend also has existed in health care—voluntary agencies that have set standards for the health care industry. These agencies and their standards are highly regarded, and their accreditation of a facility often is evidence that the facility places high priority on safety and health.

Voluntary agencies were established to enhance patient care and to ensure that the facility is a safe environment for its inhabitants. Moreover, many governmental agencies look to these voluntary groups for technical assistance in developing regulations for the health care industry. When incorporated into federal, state, or local regulations, voluntary standards become compulsory.

The JCAHO, the NFPA, the American National Standards Institute (ANSI), and the Compressed Gas Association (CGA) represent just a few of the many helpful voluntary organizations. Trade groups exist for practically every health care facility safety topic imaginable, and many states or regions have their own health care associations. Health care facilities are urged to make use of the many professional resources available to them. (See appendix A for a brief list of suggested organizations.)

Joint Commission on Accreditation of Healthcare Organizations

With the growth of the voluntary compliance movement, regional and national health care associations appeared across the country. In 1951, several of these groups, including the American Hospital Association (AHA) and the American Medical Association (AMA), founded the Joint Commission on Accreditation of Healthcare Organizations (JCAHO). The purpose of the JCAHO is to standardize practices and ensure at least a minimum standard for the quality of care for patients in American health care facilities.

Toward these ends, the JCAHO developed an accreditation process based on surveys and compliance with standards. These standards, along with general suggestions for rendering high-quality patient care, appear in the JCAHO *Accreditation Manual for Healthcare Organizations,* which is published annually. This manual has many helpful suggestions on what should be included in an overall safety program, including accident prevention techniques, safety committee requirements, and fire safety recommendations. In developing many of its inspection criteria, the JCAHO incorporates the standards of other entities such as the EPA, OSHA, and the NFPA. Compliance with these federal rules provides the foundation for JCAHO accreditation.

Any health care facility can apply to the JCAHO for accreditation once certain preliminary requirements have been met. After the facility has paid the appropriate fees and completed the extensive preparatory materials, a JCAHO team will conduct a survey for accreditation. If most standards are met and the facility is substantially in compliance, it will receive accreditation for three years.

The entire process of accreditation can be beneficial. Facilities can avail themselves of the full consulting resources of this organization that is recognized as a source of excellence by many federal, state, and local governments. In addition, through the accreditation process, health care personnel will learn effective means of limiting risks, lowering financial losses, and improving patient care.

If seeking accreditation is not feasible, another approach is to make the guidelines found in the JCAHOs' *Accreditation Manual for Healthcare Organizations* part of the facility's comprehensive safety program. By using the manual, the facility can rely on JCAHO technical knowledge and expertise in meeting safety and health requirements.

National Fire Protection Association

The National Fire Protection Association (NFPA) is an independent, not-for-profit organization that codifies fire safety standards for the construction of all buildings in the country, including health care facilities. The organization draws on expert advice from various fields in developing its codes, and is widely recognized as a reliable source of fire protection guidance. Consequently, codes have been accepted by the federal government and many state and local governments as the basis for their fire prevention and construction codes. The JCAHO also exchanges information with the NFPA through active participation on NFPA committees.

The two most important fire safety standards for health care facilities are NFPA 99, Standard for Health Care Facilities, and NFPA 101, Life Safety Code. NFPA 99 establishes criteria for safeguarding patients and health care personnel from fire, explosion, and electrical and related hazards. (NFPA 99 is one of more than 50 NFPA publications that can be applied to health care facilities.) Subjects covered in NFPA 99 include the following:

- Safe practices in anesthetizing locations
- Piped medical gas and vacuum
- Safe use of respiratory therapy
- Essential electrical systems for health care facilities
- Safe use of electricity in patient areas of hospitals
- Health care emergency preparedness
- Laboratories

NFPA 101 establishes the codes for life safety by considering a number of elements such as early warning detection and alarm systems, fire partitions, exit identification and lighting, sprinkler systems, building care maintenance, and storage for all occupied buildings. Included in the code are requirements for emergency preparedness plans and drills, exit arrangements, portable fire extinguishers, and waste-handling systems. The disaster preparedness section provides information necessary for the preparation and implementation of a facility's individual plan.

One of the best sources of overall information on the latest developments in fire protection systems, equipment, and techniques is the latest edition of the NFPA *Fire Protection Handbook*. Also, an NFPA training film, *Fire Safety in Health Care Facilities*, provides an overview of fire protection methods. Another NFPA film, *Evacuation of Medical Facilities*, focuses on successful evacuations from health care facilities.

The NFPA also is an excellent source of training materials including books, pamphlets, posters, slide programs, films, and manuals. In addition, a number of seminars are offered each year. Technical advice also is available. An individual membership is beneficial for the person most responsible for the fire safety function in each facility.

American National Standards Institute

In 1918, several professional organizations and government agencies formed the American National Standards Institute (ANSI) to coordinate the issuance of standards by agencies with similar responsibilities. The goal of ANSI is to minimize duplication and conflict between the numerous regulations affecting business and industry. The organization works to assist voluntary and government agencies in developing regulations or guidelines while seeking consensus on the need for such standards.

ANSI conducts a review process by which a regulation or requirement is approved as an American National Standard. To achieve this approval, the agency issuing the standard must be able to provide evidence that all those affected by the standard were allowed to either participate in or comment on the development of the standard. With this approval, the standard is then generally recognized and accepted for use. ANSI approval extends to regulations affecting health care as well, such as the safe use of medical lasers.

Compressed Gas Association

Health care facilities routinely use a number of compressed gases, including ethylene oxide, anesthetic gases, and oxygen. Because these gases are stored under tremendous pressure, even minimal disturbance can cause this pressure to be released in a destructive manner. If not handled and stored with great caution, compressed gases pose a serious danger of explosion, fire, injury, and property damage.

The Compressed Gas Association (CGA) was founded in 1913 as a not-for-profit trade association representing the compressed gas industries. It provides technical advice and safety coordination for businesses in these industries. However, the CGA also is concerned with the handling of compressed gases wherever they are used, including health care facilities. The CGA provides a variety of services to users of compressed gases, including technical publications and audiovisual materials, and it advises the NFPA in developing compressed gas standards. The CGA is an excellent source of information on the safe use of compressed gases.

☐ Guidelines for Regulatory Inspections

Sooner or later, a health care facility will be faced with an inspection by a federal, state, or local regulatory agency. Typically, these inspections are time-consuming but need not be traumatic if advance preparations have been made by the facility. Inspections can be unannounced or announced, depending on the agency. In the case of OSHA, most inspections are conducted without advance notice. In fact, alerting an employer in advance of an unannounced OSHA inspection can bring a criminal fine of up to $1,000 and/or a six-month jail term.

Prior to the inspection, there is an opening conference with facility representatives in which the inspector provides information on the reasons for the inspection. Following the opening conference, the inspection tour takes place followed by a closing conference. The closing conference provides the opportunity for the inspector to explain what has been found and allows time for questions and answers.

Each facility should develop policies and procedures for dealing with inspections. Once the procedures are developed, all employees who might be involved in an inspection should be trained. Because OSHA and other agencies can hold an unannounced inspection at any time of the day or night, a thorough analysis of who should be trained is necessary so that the inspection can be carried out in a smooth and professional manner. A call list should be developed containing names of the individuals to be notified upon the arrival of the inspector. The following guidelines should be included in the development of an inspection procedure.

Prior to the Opening Conference

Inspectors should be greeted as promptly as possible and made comfortable. Their identification should be requested and, if appropriate, so should copies of any warrants or supporting documents. It is important to ensure that the inspector is at the correct facility. If not, assistance and directions should be offered if requested. It is important to ask if the inspection is for the entire facility or for a specific area. This information can be used to inform individuals on the call list as quickly as possible prior to the actual inspection.

Opening Conference

The reason for the inspection and the estimated time required should be determined in detail. The facility should be prepared to furnish requested information but should not supply information that is not requested.

The Inspection

Inspectors should not be left alone at any time as they may become lost or enter a hazardous area. During the inspection, the inspector and those employees who accompany the inspector should wear required personal protective equipment and observe all safety rules. Areas that are not specifically on the inspection route should not be entered. An employee should be sent ahead to areas to be inspected to ensure that someone in the area is available to assist in the inspection. Notes should be taken of everything that is said, the exact area inspected, employees interviewed, and comments made. If the inspector takes photographs, duplicates of the exact photographs taken by the inspector also should be taken and the time, date, and location of each photograph noted. If the inspector makes a videotape, consideration should be given to having a facility representative videotape the same areas. When answering questions, only pertinent information should be offered. An inspector's opinion should not be requested about an unrelated safety concern. Above all, it is important to remain friendly and cooperative.

The inspection should be prepared for in advance. For example, personal protective equipment must be available for the inspector and those who accompany the inspector. A camera, film, and keys to locked areas also should be available. Finally, as is the case for all procedures, practice inspections with employees on all shifts will help ensure a smooth inspection that will add to the integrity of the facility.

The Closing Conference

At the end of the inspection, the inspector will normally request a closing conference. A designated member of management should be informed that the closing conference is being held so that he or she can attend. Others who may contribute information needed by the inspector also may be invited. After the closing conference, the inspector should be asked for a copy of the report that will be issued. Finally, the facility should prepare a detailed report of the closing conference, including all notes, photographs, and names of employees interviewed. Additionally, the report should include a summary of any information the inspector may have given during the inspection.

☐ Conclusion

The voluntary standards and government regulations affecting health care are numerous and diverse. Most compliance organizations work to make information and assistance available to those who need it. Many regulatory officials realize their standards may seem confusing and therefore try to enhance understanding through publications, training, and direct mailings. These agencies may be contacted by mail or telephone with questions or concerns, and many agencies operate hot lines on specific topics. (See figure 2-4 for a list of the agencies discussed in this chapter and the scope of their services.) Concerned personnel who take the time to use the many resources available will find the regulations less intimidating and compliance an achievable goal.

Figure 2-4. Summary of Agencies and Their Scope

Governmental Agency	Scope
1. Occupational Safety and Health Administration (OSHA)	Workplace safety and health
2. U.S. Environmental Protection Agency (EPA)	Control of the release of harmful materials into the environment
3. Centers for Disease Control and Prevention (CDC)	Control and prevention of disease
4. U.S. Food and Drug Administration (FDA)	Supervision of the development, testing, and monitoring of food, drugs, and medical devices
5. U.S. Nuclear Regulatory Commission (NRC)	The handling, use, and disposal of radiological materials
6. State and local agencies	Workers' compensation, public health, civil rights protection for disabled people; many areas also covered by federal agencies

Voluntary Agency	Scope
1. Joint Commission on Accreditation of Healthcare Organizations (JCAHO)	Standardization of practices to ensure high-quality patient care; accreditation
2. National Fire Protection Association (NFPA)	Prevention of fire through standards and technical support
3. American National Standards Institute (ANSI)	Coordination and approval of standards
4. Compressed Gas Association (CGA)	Provision of services to users of compressed gases

Building an Effective Safety Committee

T he anatomy of a safety program can be viewed in much the same way as that of the human body. Policies and procedures are the structure and skeleton that provide the program's shape and support; and people are the muscles and tendons that move it forward. In many respects, the safety committee acts as the eyes, ears, and other senses by receiving and processing information and providing oversight and direction.

This chapter explains the role of the safety committee within the health care facility and describes its principal functions. It also describes the responsibilities of the safety director and those of the safety committee's various components—chairperson, secretary, and members.

☐ Safety Committee

The purpose of the safety committee is to enable the health care facility to maintain a safe work environment. The committee accomplishes this by monitoring and guiding the implementation, development, and evaluation processes for all safety and health functions within the institution. The committee also serves as an advisory resource for the safety director, the chief executive officer (CEO), and the facility's various administrators. Without oversight from the safety committee, the direction and quality of the facility's safety program would be seriously jeopardized.

The need for safety committees is recognized and encouraged by a number of governmental and voluntary regulatory agencies, including the Occupational Safety and Health Administration (OSHA), the Joint Commission on Accreditation of Healthcare Organizations (JCAHO), and state and local government agencies. The JCAHO not only requires facilities to have safety committees but also specifies certain duties that the committees must carry out.

The safety committee receives authority from the facility's board and CEO and is empowered to (1) make recommendations to all levels of management and (2) take necessary corrective action to achieve safety goals. Additionally, the committee is responsible for issuing identified safety management issues and summaries of safety committee activities to the board, CEO, department heads, and other individuals as appropriate.

The safety committee also serves as a catalyst to spark an active interest in safety among employees. By including both employees and managers, the safety committee can draw on their common goal of reducing employee exposure to injury. In addition to helping the committee effectively implement necessary changes in safety policies and procedures, this united effort between employees and management will allow everyone to have an important role in safety and will encourage employees to convey their enthusiasm to their coworkers. As other employees have a chance to sit on the committee, commitment to safety concerns and the willingness to actively participate will spread throughout the facility. This consequence is vital, for it is the employees' support and involvement that contribute most to the success of safety programs. By carrying out its responsibilities in a professional and effective manner, the safety committee will be viewed by both employees and management as a valuable and respected resource.

□ Safety Director

The JCAHO requires that the CEO or a designee appoint a safety director who is qualified by experience or education to develop, implement, and monitor the safety management program. In small facilities, the safety director function may be an additional task assigned to another position, such as the security director, the infection control manager, or the human resource director. In some cases, another title may be used, for example, safety manager or safety officer. Some facilities have decentralized the safety management function by making all department heads responsible for safety within their departments. In this case, the JCAHO requires that the facility must be able to establish accountability equivalent to that required when JCAHO's PTSM standard specifies a single head of the safety function.

The individual designated to carry out the safety director function must have a clear understanding of the responsibilities involved. The safety director is required to manage an ongoing facilitywide safety process, which involves the collection and evaluation of information about hazards and safety practices. The resulting information is then used to identify safety management issues to be addressed by the safety committee.

Depending on facility size, the safety director function can be defined broadly to include the roles of teacher, strategist, motivator, analyst, consultant, and regulatory expert. To perform this broad function, he or she has a number of specific responsibilities, including any or all of the following:

- Establishing indicators that monitor events such as fire drills and safety surveys, and taking action when those indicators have been exceeded
- Helping establish facilitywide and department-specific safety policies by serving as consultant and sounding board for various department managers who are writing the policies
- Managing the collection and analysis of information such as hazard surveillance surveys, incident reports, and other monitoring data
- Providing the safety committee with information summaries that will enable it to take appropriate action
- Participating, where appropriate, in the safety incident investigation and reporting process
- Participating in the selection and design of employee orientation and continuing education programs
- Providing the safety committee with expertise and direction
- Acting as liaison between the safety committee and other committees such as radiation, laser safety, and infection control
- Maintaining safety records, ensuring that proper documentation is kept and that corrective action on major safety problems is taken in a timely manner

The safety director also must respond to safety problems and often is called on to make decisions that require immediate action. This responsibility should be part of the authority given the safety director by the CEO. To ensure that the safety director's authority is understood facilitywide, his or her appointment should be publicized and an announcement made that he or she has been granted authority to make decisions affecting the safety of the employees and the facility.

□ Safety Committee Composition

The safety committee is composed essentially of three components: chairperson, secretary, and members. The following subsections describe the functions and responsibilities of each of these components.

Committee Chairperson

The overall direction of the safety committee rests with the chairperson. This individual must be capable of providing strong leadership and must possess good interpersonal skills and management capability. The chairperson also must be knowledgeable in safety and preferably have experience serving on a safety committee. In some facilities, the committee chairperson position is filled by the safety director. However, such an arrangement may not always be advisable because it may centralize safety decision making to the extent that a full range of ideas and alternatives is not always considered.

In addition to overall management of the safety committee, the chairperson is responsible for the following:

- Developing a meeting schedule
- Arranging a place to convene
- Notifying members of meetings
- Planning meeting agendas
- Reviewing the minutes and materials for the meeting
- Obtaining any speakers or instructors for the meeting
- Leading and facilitating discussion during the meeting
- Publicizing safety committee activities and successes throughout the facility
- Developing a process for educating new members about the committee's functions and structure

Some facilities rotate the chairperson position every year to increase participation and avoid burnout. The practice of rotation affords a greater number of people the opportunity to contribute and bring new ideas to the safety program. However, some large facilities have taken the position that frequent rotation leads to a weaker committee because of the loss of experience needed to manage a complex program. Rotation should be carefully managed to avoid this problem.

Committee Secretary

To expedite committee activities and maintain necessary documentation, the committee should have a secretary. The secretary should be experienced, with a demonstrated desire to participate in safety matters. In some facilities, he or she is responsible for performing the following tasks:

- Preparing and distributing committee meeting agenda and minutes
- Documenting the status of committee recommendations
- Preparing and distributing meeting materials
- Assisting the chairperson, as requested

Committee Members

In addition to the secretary and the chairperson, the safety committee must have representation from several departments and levels in the facility hierarchy. Depending on facility size, safety committee members may include the following:

- Administration representative
- Medical staff representative

- Nursing representative(s)
- Director of maintenance (or engineering, or both)
- Supervisory representatives (one or two on rotation)
- Director of housekeeping
- Director of dietary
- Human resources representative
- Safety director
- Security director
- Labor representative (if applicable)
- Risk management representative
- Three nonsupervisory caregivers

The goal in selecting committee members is to provide a multidisciplinary committee. Although the JCAHO does not specify the exact composition of the committee, commission accreditation surveyors do look for a committee with representation from the administration, clinical, and support services. (See figure 3-1 for a graphic representation of this multidisciplinary approach.) Larger facilities may expand on this minimum membership and include representatives from departments such as infection control, quality assurance, employee health, and pathology.

Committee size should be limited to approximately 15 members. Too many members can cause the group to become unwieldy and unproductive. To avoid the pitfalls of one excessively large committee, some facilities adopt a multilayered structure. This structure utilizes subcommittees, each with a clearly defined set of responsibilities. The subcommittees report to the safety committee on a scheduled basis. (See figure 3-2 for a typical reporting schedule for a large facility.) The reporting schedules should be developed and published annually so that subcommittees can prepare well in advance.

Member rotation can be a valuable process for the same reasons as those for chairperson rotation. Rotation brings new ideas and fresh motivation from new members. It also gives

Figure 3-1. The Multidisciplinary Safety Committee

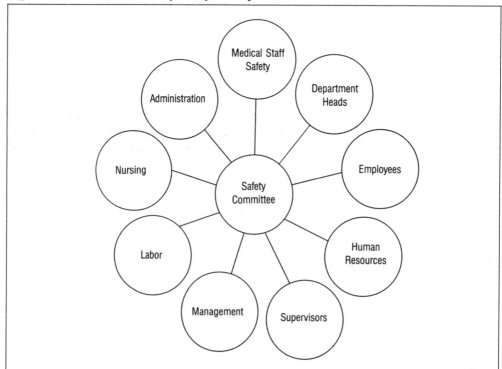

Figure 3-2. Safety Committee Reporting Schedule

Subcommittee Reports to the Safety Committee

	Jan.	Feb.	Mar.	Apr.	May	June	July	Aug.	Sept.	Oct.	Nov.	Dec.
Emergency Response		X			X			X			X	
Equipment/Utilities		X			X			X			X	
Infection Control			X			X		X		X		X
Life Safety			X			X			X			X
Loss Prevention			X			X			X			X
Quality Assurance		X		X		X		X		X		X
Radiation Safety	X			X			X			X		

Safety Committee Reports to the Facility

	Jan.	Feb.	Mar.	Apr.	May	June	July	Aug.	Sept.	Oct.	Nov.	Dec.
Safety Report to Hospital QA												X
Safety Program Report to Board of Trustees			X			X			X			X
Safety Program Report to Department Heads	X			X			X			X		

Reprinted, with permission, from Lehigh Valley Hospital, Allentown, PA.

administrative and operational employees a better understanding of, and commitment to, safety. However, because of the increasing complexity of regulatory requirements, care must be exercised to avoid loss of technical expertise. In any case, the rotation of members should be staggered to ensure that the committee's composition includes experienced members at all times.

Member responsibilities need to be clarified in any group setting, and new safety committee members should be trained in their individual responsibilities as well as those of the committee as a body. New member training should occur as soon as possible after assignment. It is important to let new members know that they were chosen because the organization values their knowledge and capabilities.

Although member responsibilities vary widely depending on facility size and type, they normally include the following:

- Providing two-way communication between the committee and the facility personnel they represent
- Participating in incident investigations and safety inspections
- Contributing ideas and suggestions for improvement
- Acting as models of sound safety practices for other employees
- Reporting exemplary employee behavior
- Placing a high priority on attendance and actively participating in committee programs

Figure 3-3 summarizes the basic responsibilities of safety committee participants.

Labor-Management Cooperation

Both labor and management have the same safety goal of reducing employee exposure to injury. Safety committees can draw on this common goal by including labor and management

Figure 3-3. Responsibilities of Safety Committee Participants

Chairperson

- Schedule meetings.
- Arrange location.
- Notify members.
- Plan agenda.
- Prepare for meeting.
- Obtain any necessary speakers.
- Lead discussion.
- Publicize committee activities.
- Educate new members.

Secretary

- Prepare minutes and agenda.
- Distribute minutes.
- Document status of committee recommendations.
- Prepare and distribute meeting materials.
- Assist the chairperson.

Members

- Provide information from the committee to the facility personnel they represent.
- Provide feedback to the committee from the personnel they represent.
- Participate in incident investigations and safety inspections.
- Contribute ideas and suggestions for improvement.
- Act as models of sound safety practices for other employees.
- Report exemplary employee behavior.
- Place a high priority on attendance and actively participate in committee programs.

representatives on the safety committee. A united effort between labor and management can help the safety committee effectively implement necessary changes in safety policies and procedures.

When a joint safety committee with both management and labor representation is established, the chairperson should stress that members have much to gain from effective cooperation. The committee is not an arena in which differences are to be debated but, rather, one in which safety issues are to be discussed. Additionally, to prevent disputes, the chairperson should ensure that labor and management members do not participate in contract negotiations while serving on the committee. This way, the committee is buffered from the collective bargaining process.

As with other committee participants, members must be chosen who are highly motivated toward making the workplace safer and more healthful. As the combined safety committee members begin to perceive mutual objectives and assess the overall safety program, they will realize the value of being involved in such a bilateral effort. Members will take measurable steps toward understanding one another better, while learning from each other along the way.

☐ Safety Committee Functions

The primary function of the safety committee is to monitor the effectiveness of the facility's safety programs and activities and to assist in complying with regulatory and voluntary agency requirements. Therefore, the committee must establish a process that provides information from all safety programs and activities. Because of the volume of safety information generated, the information must be presented or available in a form that can be used effectively by the committee.

The amount of information the committee must process depends on the size of the facility. A multisite research facility with 600 beds can generate substantially more information than a small two-story rural facility. These two facilities require safety committees with different structures and management skills. However, the primary function of both committees is the same, and many of the same safety issues must be addressed using similar processes. Only the number and complexity of the programs are different.

However, regardless of facility size, the committee is expected to manage the following tasks:

- Ensure that the facility's safety information management process defines, obtains, analyzes, and reports information in a manner that allows and supports timely safety management decisions

- Require the use of indicators for assessing safety performance, processes, and outcomes
- Review and evaluate all required facilitywide and department-specific reports
- Use a process to resolve identified safety concerns and assign specific safety tasks to appropriate individuals or subcommittees for remedial action
- Issue quarterly reports of safety management issues and safety committee activities to the governing body, the CEO, department heads, and others responsible for safety monitoring activities
- Establish strategies to enable the facility to comply with JCAHO provisions, as well as the requirements of relevant government and voluntary agencies
- Evaluate the feasibility and effectiveness of corrective action plans and monitor them until completed
- Review and approve all safety policies and procedures prior to adoption and annually thereafter
- Assess the facility's safety programs annually, including identifying deficiencies and the status of performance improvement activities

The information required to carry out these functions comes from a number of sources, depending on facility size. In some cases, the information is provided in a summarized report from subcommittees, including the following:

- Emergency management
- Equipment and utilities
- Loss prevention
- Radiation safety
- Waste management
- Laser safety
- Life safety
- Occupational health
- Infection control
- Security
- Risk management

The safety committee uses information from the subcommittees to carry out the functions described above. Figure 3-4 shows a multilayered safety structure that may be required in a large facility.

Other sources of information may be routinely required by the safety committee. For example, employee training information is provided by the human resource department or specific training committees. Additionally, the safety director and individual department heads provide the committee with summaries and trend data on injuries, incidents, and hazard surveillance. In small facilities that do not use subcommittees, information comes from individuals who are responsible for the management of specific safety issues.

In order to effectively manage corrective action programs, the committee should maintain a tracking system. Following are some of the elements that should be included:

- Date the item (injury, incident, hazard) was reported
- Planned corrective action
- Responsibility for action
- Status of action
- Completion date(s)

The status of "items due" should be reviewed by the committee at each meeting. During this review, the committee plays an important role in identifying and removing roadblocks and completing corrective action items on schedule. (See figure 12-8, p. 136, for a typical corrective action tracking form.)

Figure 3-4. Safety Committee Organization

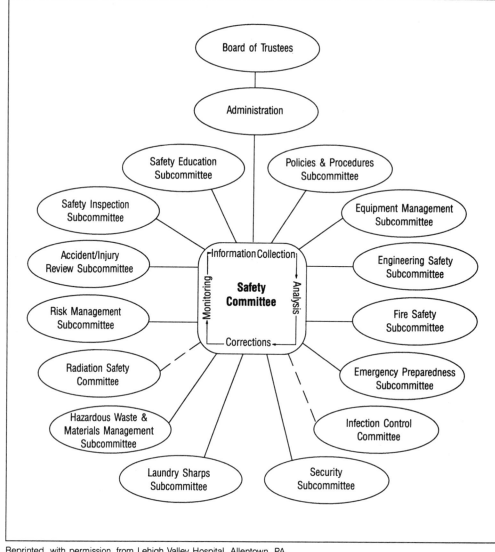

Reprinted, with permission, from Lehigh Valley Hospital, Allentown, PA.

The JCAHO requires that safety committee recommendations and actions be reported at least quarterly to administration, the board, managers of departments/services, and others as appropriate. The facility must be able to provide evidence that these recommendations and actions are implemented and the effectiveness of changes are monitored. Follow-up action and results of monitoring must be reported to the safety committee and documented in safety committee minutes.

Task Forces

Many committees use a task force to deal with a specific safety issue. This is an effective method for accomplishing short-term safety objectives. The task force can be dissolved upon completion of the assignment. For example, in a facility in which equipment failures have increased in a number of areas and are causing alarm, a task force of two or three employees knowledgeable about the equipment can be assigned to investigate specific failures. Each task force then documents its activities and reports back to the safety committee.

Committee Meetings

The most frequently asked question on the topic of safety committees is, How can meetings be more effective? Most employees easily grasp committee composition, goals, and functions but find improving meeting effectiveness a difficult problem. Frustration with committees is natural. In fact, committees are notorious for their inefficiency and their members' corresponding lack of enthusiasm.

Lengthy and disorganized meetings are symptomatic of a poorly managed safety committee. Meetings usually are most successful when held once a month for no longer than an hour. Lengthy meetings can be corrected by good preplanning on the part of the chairperson and subcommittee leaders. For example, members should be asked to contact the chairperson well in advance of the meeting if they want something placed on the agenda. Once the agenda has been determined, the chairperson should send it to members at least one week in advance of the meeting. This serves to alert members that a meeting is approaching. Supporting documentation, such as inspection results and the minutes of the previous meeting, should be distributed with the agenda. (See figure 3-5 for a sample agenda.) Additionally, it is helpful to publish a calendar of meeting times, dates, and places at the beginning of the year so that members can schedule their time and make their preparations accordingly.

There are other ways to add to the success of meetings. The meeting room should be large enough to easily accommodate everyone, and should be comfortable, private, and free of distractions. Using the same site for every meeting will heighten members' comfort in familiar surroundings.

Another approach is to occasionally vary the format by inviting knowledgeable and entertaining speakers. This way, the committee learns while getting a break from its routine work. Additionally, members should be rewarded for their efforts. For example, refreshments and occasional appreciation lunches encourage member participation. A little pampering often goes a long way.

Figure 3-5. Sample Safety Committee Agenda

Date:

Time:

Place:

1. Roll call (list those present).
2. Reading of minutes from previous meeting.
3. Unfinished business from previous meeting.
4. Closure of any previous business (describe).
5. Discussion of new business; topics could include:*

   - Inspection reports
   - Reports on safety training
   - Incident trends and serious incidents
   - Outstanding recommendations
   - Evaluation of program effectiveness
   - A speaker
   - Revisions of safety policies and procedures
   - Other safety concerns of the facility
   - Incentive programs planned

6. Goal setting.
7. Date and time of next meeting.
8. Adjournment

*To allow adequate time for discussion, only one or two topics should be discussed at each meeting.

How well the safety committee performs depends in large part on the performance of the committee chairperson. For example, he or she should avoid taking an excessively demanding approach to members. It is important to remember that members are volunteering valuable time and effort to the program. In addition, the chairperson should facilitate and not monopolize discussion. And finally, he or she should acknowledge member contributions during the meetings. By planning properly, following a consistent format, and making an effort to motivate members, the chairperson can do a great deal to enhance committee effectiveness.

☐ Conclusion

Safety committees can serve as a valuable resource and advisory group promoting and advancing safety. The key to success is organizing the committee and its functions, balancing representation, and motivating and rewarding its members. Reevaluating and perhaps restructuring the facility's existing committee can provide numerous benefits. Whatever the status of the present committee, a renewed interest in conducting more successful meetings can boost performance. With some time and attention invested in this group, the safety committee can become an effective force that sustains and guides a results-oriented safety program.

Departmental Safety

Although the facilitywide safety program forms a coordinated, integrated whole, safety also must be implemented at the departmental level. It is here that employees carry out the program's requirements and procedures. At this level, safe actions and preventive measures, outlined in specific departmental policies and procedures, have the greatest impact on the overall success of the safety program. Many departments have similar safety concerns that can be approached using basic safety concepts common to all such risks.

This chapter provides an overview of hazards present in clinical and support services. It also discusses various types of personal protective equipment.

☐ Safety in Clinical Services

Clinical services are those departments or areas directly involved in patient care—for example, nursing, anesthesiology, and pathology. Such services encounter problems in patient care delivery that may not directly affect support services. The following subsections describe many of these clinical service areas and the hazards most likely to occur in them. Also included is a discussion of safety considerations required when handling two specific materials commonly used in clinical areas.

Patient Care Areas

In patient care areas, the most frequently reported types of occupational injury are strains and sprains. Tasks such as lifting patients and moving beds and heavy materials are primary contributors to the frequency of such injuries. (See chapter 5 for a discussion of measures that can help prevent strains and sprains.)

Cuts, lacerations, and punctures also are common among health care workers in clinical care areas. These injuries often occur because of improper disposal of needles and other sharp items. The Occupational Safety and Health Administration (OSHA) Bloodborne Pathogens Standard (1910.1030) (see chapter 7) requires engineering and work practice controls to avoid needle sticks and cuts.

Chemotherapy drugs create additional hazards for employees who administer them. Employees must be trained in the use of preventive measures to reduce the risk of exposure to these substances during patient care. (See chapter 6 for a discussion of precautions required in administering these drugs.)

Surgical Services, Dialysis, and Special Care Units

A primary concern in surgery, as well as in dialysis and special care units, is electrical safety. Sophisticated electrical equipment must be used, with no margin for error. A number of electrical safety measures can be taken to ensure employee safety. These include:

- A system of preventive maintenance should be established whereby all electrical equipment is inspected regularly and maintained constantly to prevent hazards. The Joint Commission on Accreditation of Healthcare Organizations (JCAHO) requires specific inspection programs for patient-use and nonpatient-use equipment.
- Frayed electrical cords, or those with deteriorated insulation, should be replaced.
- Electrical cords should be secured and kept out of high-traffic areas to avoid tripping hazards.
- Electrical equipment must be properly grounded or double-insulated.
- The facility must comply with NFPA 101 (Life Safety Code for the National Fire Protection Association).
- Electrical equipment, appliances, or wall receptacles that appear to be damaged should be repaired before use.
- Electrical safety training should be provided, where appropriate.
- Emergency power generators must be tested and maintained to provide electricity to crucial life support and life safety equipment during interruption of the normal electrical source.

Anesthesiology

Special care should be taken to ensure the safe administration of anesthetic gases. Written safety procedures must be established to minimize electrical hazards. If flammable agents are used, all sources of ignition or explosion should be removed. In addition, personnel must be protected from excessive exposure to anesthetizing agents, which may cause adverse health effects. Effective gas-scavenging systems should be instituted, along with regularly scheduled maintenance of anesthesia equipment, to prevent leakage.

Respiratory Therapy

Oxygen fires constitute the foremost threat in respiratory therapy. Signage must be used to indicate areas where oxygen is in use, and smoking must be prohibited in these areas. Electrical equipment that could generate sparks or raise the temperature substantially should be prohibited.

In addition to the hazard posed by oxygen, respiratory workers face three other potential hazards. One hazard is the high risk of exposure to patients with tuberculosis (TB) and other airborne diseases. (See chapter 11 for a discussion of OSHA recommendations for protecting employees against the spread of TB.) A second hazard is exposure to airborne drugs during patient treatment. Because some of these drugs can have serious side effects, appropriate protective measures such as respirators and ventilation should be used. A third hazard is exposure to blood and body fluids, especially when suctioning or inducing a cough response. To prevent such exposure, protective gear should be worn and applicable safety measures met.

Radiology and Nuclear Medicine

It is imperative that the radiology and nuclear medicine departments have written policies and procedures for the safe use, storage, and disposal of radiological materials. These procedures must satisfy requirements of the Nuclear Regulatory Commission (NRC). These requirements include limiting the exposure of employees to radiation, actions to be taken after accidental exposure, appropriate use of caution signs, personal radiation dosimeters, and record keeping.

X-ray machines can emit dangerous levels of radiation and must be used carefully. The reproductive systems of patients and technicians should be shielded and kept at a protective distance from the source of radiation at all times. In addition, adequate protection should be provided for employees working around implant patients because implants also may give off high levels of radiation. Those employees at risk of being affected by radiation include personnel from nursing, housekeeping, radiology, and pathology.

Pathology

All hazardous materials and wastes from the pathology department must be handled according to applicable regulations and guidelines. The OSHA Laboratory Standard (29 CFR 1910.1200) specifies that a chemical hygiene plan must be developed that outlines measures to be taken to protect employees against hazardous chemicals. Some of the more common chemicals found in pathology include formaldehyde, glutaraldehyde, and xylene. OSHA regulations require monitoring to ensure that safe levels are maintained. (See figure 4-1 for a summary of laboratory safety precautions used in pathology.)

Emergency Department

The emergency department (ED) frequently is the busiest department in the hospital. Often patients and relatives are in a distracted state, which can be exacerbated by long waits. Security must be adequate in EDs, and emergency staff should work to calm visitors. Staff members who may have contact with blood, including those who clean up spills of blood, must be adequately protected against bloodborne infectious diseases.

Emergency department employees also are exposed to possible violent behavior of patients and other individuals who come to the department. One informal study in five California metropolitan area EDs showed that 40 percent of 103 managers reported physical threats to staff 5 to 15 times per month. Training in intervention procedures should be given to all ED employees.

Figure 4-1. Laboratory Safety Precautions

- Observe rules for infectious agents and toxic substances.
- Walk carefully. Floors in lab areas where paraffin is used are extremely slippery.
- Wash hands often with disinfectant soap, and always wash before leaving the work area.
- Cleanse and dress a cut or puncture immediately and, using appropriate protocol, note the cause of injury and the material handled.
- Report any accident or injury.
- Handle all tissue samples, bloods, and serums as though they were from infected patients.
- Use all necessary personal protective equipment (such as a face mask and/or surgical latex or other appropriate gloves) when handling infectious materials.
- Wash hands thoroughly after handling hazardous or infectious materials, even if gloves were worn.
- Put all hazardous material in labeled plastic bags or other appropriate container for disposal.
- Use both hands when handling large bottles and never lift bottles by the top alone.
- Use a mechanical pipette aid to draw material into a pipette. Never use the mouth to suck any material into a pipette.
- Remove all broken glass from countertops to prevent slivers from cutting hands, arms, and elbows.
- Discard all glassware, syringes, and needles into labeled, puncture-resistant containers for this purpose.
- Wear gloves to remove materials from ovens and autoclaves.
- Observe usage rules on all laminar flow hoods.
- Chain gas cylinders in place. Separate full cylinders from empty ones.

Pharmacy

In the pharmacy, workers are exposed to various hazards that can cause back injuries, cuts, and exposures to chemicals and drugs. The following control measures should be considered:

- Stepladders should be used to reach items stored on high shelves.
- Spills should be cleaned up promptly.
- Broken bottles and unusable pharmaceuticals should be disposed of according to established procedures.
- Adequate fume hoods should be provided in areas where prescriptions and chemotherapeutic drugs are mixed or ground.

To prevent improper dispensing, drugs should be labeled with the patient's full name and room number. Stock should be inspected regularly, and outdated drugs should be disposed of properly. Cytotoxic drugs should be handled cautiously, according to relevant guidelines (see chapter 6).

Special Safety Programs in Clinical Areas

Two particular materials used in the hospital's clinical areas require development of specific safety programs. These materials are lasers and compressed gas.

Laser Safety Program

The term *laser* is an acronym for light amplification by stimulated emission of radiation. Lasers often are considered preferable to scalpels because they can eliminate extensive bleeding. They have a wide variety of surgical uses, including gynecological, general, plastic, and eye surgeries. However, they also generate dangerous nonionizing radiation, create hazards to vision, and give off smoke and fumes.

The laser safety program should include procedures to train and protect all potentially affected personnel including staff nurses, operating room technicians, physicians, anesthesia staff, and laser support personnel. All personnel involved in the use of lasers should take part in a medical surveillance program to prevent eye damage. Both affected personnel and patients should wear appropriate eye protection, and a warning sign should be used when the laser is in operation. A program of preventive maintenance for laser equipment also should be in place.

Smoke created during laser use can be irritating and dangerous, and should be evacuated using a commercial smoke evacuator. Additionally, the evacuated smoke should be filtered before it is exhausted from the building.

Compressed Gas Safety Program

Health care facilities use a variety of compressed gases, including oxygen, nitrous oxide, and ethylene oxide (EtO). Gases such as oxygen and nitrous oxide support combustion, whereas gases such as propane and acetylene are considered flammable.

Because these gases are stored under extreme pressure, care must be taken to ensure that the gas tanks are properly secured to prevent them from accidentally tipping over and damaging the valve. Valve failure could result in an extremely dangerous condition called rocketing, in which the cylinder is propelled with enough force to blast through a concrete block wall. Thus, it is imperative that the facility develop procedures for the safe handling, storage, and transport of compressed gas cylinders. When storing compressed gas cylinders, several precautions must be taken. Cylinders should be stored:

- In an upright and secured position (*Secured* usually means in a tank holder or chained to a fixed object such as a wall.)
- In designated areas only
- Away from radiators, direct sunlight, and other sources of heat

- In a well-protected, well-ventilated, dry location
- At least 20 feet from combustible materials including paper, rags, and oil or other petroleum products
- Away from elevators, stairs, or gangways
- In areas protected against being knocked over or subject to tampering by unauthorized persons

When transporting compressed gas cylinders, the cylinders must be secured to prevent damage. For example, a cylinder cart or hand truck with the chain or strap in place could be used. During transport, cylinders must not be allowed to be struck or to strike each other because the contact may cause them to rupture or fall.

Compressed gas cylinder safety involves adherence to a number of other guidelines. For example:

- Cylinders must be labeled to identify contents and hazard information.
- Cylinders must have pressure-relief devices and connections that comply with Compressed Gas Association (CGA) standards.
- Valves should be closed when cylinders are not in use.
- Defective cylinders should be returned to the supplier.

☐ Safety for Support Services

Support services are those departments that contribute to patient care indirectly. Among the areas that provide these services are administration, housekeeping, food service, engineering, and central supply. The following subsections describe the safety hazards that exist in these areas as well as two related safety considerations: construction and renovation safety and helicopter safety.

Administration

Office areas frequently are overlooked during health and safety inspections. The following guidelines should be included in a program designed for office employees:

- Use of extension cords should be discouraged because they may cause employees to trip and fall. Temporary electrical cords and telephone cables that cross aisles should be taped to the floor or covered with material designed to anchor them.
- All uncarpeted floors should have antislip surfaces. Stumbling hazards such as frayed carpet and loose tiles should be repaired.
- Aisles and passageways must be kept clear to avoid fire hazards and tripping.
- Adequate ventilation should be provided around office equipment that uses chemicals, and employees must be informed of the hazards involved and taught how to protect themselves. (See chapter 6 for a discussion of methods for reducing exposure to chemicals.)
- Ergonomic chairs should be provided when needed. These chairs should be equipped with casters that are specifically designed for carpet or tile.
- Heavy materials should not be stored on high shelves.
- Desks and countertops should be free of sharp, square corners.

Housekeeping

Because they work in all patient and nonpatient areas, housekeeping employees are potentially exposed to all of the health and safety hazards found in the facility. In many areas, strictly aseptic conditions must be maintained at all times. Thus, housekeeping personnel must be well trained in ensuring that these conditions exist. Following are guidelines that should be included in a program for housekeeping employees:

- Training should include the safe use of electrical power equipment, especially electrical scrub machines and other cleaning equipment that will be used with or around water. (See figure 4-2 for a general list of equipment safety measures for all health care facility services.)
- Light bulbs should be changed carefully, not when they are hot or when someone is underneath them.
- Electrical equipment should be disconnected from the power source before it is cleaned.
- Cleaning agents proven to be toxic to human health, highly flammable, or explosive should be replaced with less dangerous materials whenever possible.
- Employees must be informed about the hazardous chemicals they work with and be trained in their safe use. Chemicals are frequently used by housekeeping employees, including soaps and detergents, solvents, cleaners, and disinfectants.
- Employees should be aware that other persons may not have followed proper procedures for disposing of needles, knives, and glassware. All refuse should be handled as if hazardous items were present.
- Slippery areas on floors that are being scrubbed or polished should be identified with signs or should be roped off.

Food Service

In food service areas, many injuries can occur as a result of wet and greasy floors, faulty food-processing equipment, and the handling, receiving, processing, and distribution of materials. These hazards can be eliminated by training employees to correctly handle materials, properly guard machinery and hot surfaces, maintain dry and orderly walking and working surfaces, and implement good housekeeping practices. There are a number of ways to reduce these hazards. For example:

- Electrical components and equipment should be serviced routinely.
- Employees should be trained in correct materials-handling techniques.
- Machinery and hot surfaces should be guarded properly.
- Dry, uncluttered walking and working surfaces should be maintained.
- Good work and housekeeping practices should be maintained.

Figure 4-2. General Equipment Safety Measures

- Read the instructions that accompany a new piece of equipment before using it.
- Carry portable equipment, such as a mop or broom, close to the body to avoid injuring anyone.
- Station equipment out of the way. Never permit equipment to block exits, fire doors, fire extinguisher or fire hose cabinets, stairwells, or elevators.
- Clean equipment after use. Turn buckets upside down to dry thoroughly. Mops and cleaning cloths should be changed with each shift.
- Keep equipment in good repair, for example, nuts and bolts tight, broken parts repaired or replaced.
- Report broken equipment immediately, remove it from service, and label the equipment as defective until repaired. Do not put broken equipment in a storage area containing operable equipment.
- Make sure electrical equipment is in working order and is grounded when in use. Do not use adapters. When using electrical rotary cleaning machines on wet floors, make sure all wiring and connections are sound.
- Wear rubber-soled shoes or rubber slipovers to prevent slipping.
- Do not clean ramps with power equipment.
- Make sure an adequate number of various sizes and types of ladders are available and in good repair. Set ladders firmly in position, and never stand on the top two rungs or steps. Do not use chairs, tables, or other furniture as stools or ladders.

A number of other safety precautions should be taken. For example:

- Floors must be promptly cleaned of spills, and employees should wear shoes with non-skid soles.
- Glass and china should be stored safely and conveniently.
- Employees should be trained in the safe handling of knives and other cutting equipment.
- Employees should keep glassware separate from metal utensils and wash knives individually and carefully, when washing dishes in a sink.
- For prevention of burns:
  —Potholders should be abundant and accessible.
  —Hot foods should be poured away from the body.
  —Handles of pots and pans should be turned away from the edge of the range.
  —Minor burns should be treated immediately by soaking them in cold water or applying ice.

In addition to safety hazards posed to employees, poor food sanitation practices can create health hazards. Good sanitary practices include proper food storage and temperature control. Pesticides should be applied only by trained personnel and should not be allowed to contaminate food. (Effective pest control includes cleanup and proper storage of food.) Additionally, regular handwashing should be required of all dietary personnel. (See figure 4-3 for a list of general sanitation and personal hygiene measures.)

Food service employee clothing and hairstyles must be in accordance with federal and state regulations. Figure 4-4 suggests protective clothing for food service and other support services staff.

Engineering

Maintenance shops can pose a number of dangers to employees. Following are some general guidelines for maintenance areas:

- Blade guards must be installed on motorized saws.
- Electrical equipment must be properly grounded or double-insulated.
- Extension cords must be of the three-wire type and of sufficient capacity to safely carry the required load. Additionally, extension cords may be used only in temporary locations and should not be substituted for fixed wiring.
- Equipment guards must be in use while the equipment is operating.
- Metal ladders should never be used to change light bulbs or work on electrical equipment or wiring.
- Broken ladders must be destroyed or tagged, removed from service, or repaired.
- Protective clothing and equipment must be provided for and worn by all employees exposed to hazards requiring protection. For example:
  —Gloves (for handling chemicals and hot, wet, or sharp objects)
  —Hearing protection (to prevent hearing loss from noise sources)
  —Eye and face protection (for protection from chips, sparks, glare, and splashes)
  —Respirators (to prevent exposure to hazardous and infectious materials)
- All gasoline-powered equipment must be properly maintained and only operated in well-ventilated areas to prevent the buildup of carbon monoxide.
- All hand tools must be kept in good repair and stored properly.
- Confined space entry, such as cleaning boilers and tanks, must be done following written procedures that comply with OSHA Confined Space Standard, 29 CFR 1910.146.
- All energized sources must be properly locked out during maintenance work per the OSHA Lockout/Tagout Standard, 29 CFR 1910.147.
- Care must be taken to avoid damaging cylinders during handling and storage. (See the section on Compressed Gas Safety Program on p. 36.)

Figure 4-3. General Sanitation Measures for Food Service

1. Keep all foods at safe temperatures. Bacteria grow best within the range of 50° to 140° F. Once food is prepared, it should never be allowed to remain within that temperature range. All foods ready to be served should be kept at hot (above 140° F) or cold (below 45° F) temperatures.

   Cooked foods should be brought to a temperature above the bacteria-killing level and should be maintained at that temperature until they are served. Cold foods should be kept cold until they are served.

   Defrosting should be done far enough in advance so that it can be done in a refrigerator below 45° F.

2. Follow safe techniques for cooling or reheating leftovers. Cool all leftover hot foods quickly by placing them in shallow containers in the coolest area of the refrigerator. Reheat leftovers only once, bringing them above the 140° F killing point.

3. Avoid cross-contamination. If raw and ready-to-serve foods are mixed in processing or storage, bacteria from the raw foods may contaminate the ready-to-serve foods. Do not mix these foods, because they usually cannot be heated above killing temperature.

   Cross-contamination can also occur when cutting boards, knives, and appliances are not cleaned after use and are used for both types of food. These tools should be washed following each use.

4. Store food properly. Refrigerated foods should be covered to avoid contamination brought about by foods touching each other or the shelves and walls of the refrigerator. Sanitary storage temperatures for foods are:
   a. Dry—50–70° F
   b. Chilled—45° F or less
   c. Frozen—0° F or less

5. Handle food properly. Utensils or tools should be used to handle food rather than bare hands. If food must be touched, disposable plastic gloves must be worn. Never put a tasting spoon back into the food after it has been used.

6. Clean tableware, equipment, and utensils at appropriate temperatures. Mechanical dishwasher water should remain above the bacteria-killing point of 140° F with the final rinse temperature set at 180° F. Follow the manufacturer's instructions for positioning dishes in the dishwasher. Use the appropriate detergent in the proper amount for both mechanical and hand washing. Rinse the dishwasher and clean the foodtraps following each meal. All appliances should be cleaned, sanitized, and protected against contamination.

7. Insist on good personal hygiene. Personnel must wash before beginning work, after using the restroom, and after touching any soiled item. To encourage these habits, handsoap and towels must be readily available in the kitchen and bathrooms. Bathrooms should also be kept very clean. Clean uniforms, hair nets, disposable plastic gloves, and personal protective equipment should be provided and used.

8. Have a liberal sick leave policy. Employees with sore throats, gastrointestinal infections, infected cuts, nasal discharge, burns, sores, or boils should be sent home or given other tasks to avoid infecting the people in the facility.

9. Control insects and pests. Flies may transmit up to 30 types of bacteria, including those causing typhoid, dysentery, and diarrhea. Screens in windows and doors will help keep them out, but the best control is to eliminate their breeding ground. Keep all garbage cans covered, and promptly clean up all filth and debris in and around the facility.

   Roaches are another common pest. They are attracted to dark, damp, and dirty areas, such as near sinks, around water pipes, and in corners and crevices. They carry many bacteria, including salmonella. To control roach infestation, fill all cracks and crevices, keep all food service areas clean and orderly, and inspect all incoming supplies for signs of roaches.

   Rodents are the carriers of many dangerous bacteria and, due to their size, they can destroy much food. Cracks and crevices should be filled in and around the building to keep them out. Rodenticides also help control them. Good housekeeping methods and sanitary handling and storage are a primary defense against pests. Also, consult with a pest-control service.

10. Store chemical compounds away from foods. Always be certain that cleaning and disinfectant supplies are stored in distinctive containers that are clearly marked with contents, cautions, and first-aid measures. Keep all chemicals and cleaning solutions away from bulk storage areas.

Reprinted, with permission, from National Safety Council. *Long Term Care Safety Management Manual: A Handbook for Practical Application.* Chicago: National Safety Council, 1987, pp. 36–38.

Figure 4-4. Protective Clothing for Support Services Personnel

Central Service

- Impervious gloves to eliminate skin contact with irritating chemicals.
- Respirator (when required) used only by people who are trained and in a medical surveillance/training program for respirator use.
- Chemical apron and full-face shield, when required.

Dietary

- Low-heeled shoes with slip-resistant soles and boots for wet areas.
- Impervious gloves for washing pots and pans and for consistently wet hands.
- Metal mesh gloves for meatcutters and others who use knives frequently.
- Rubber gloves and goggles or a face shield for handlers of concentrated liquid ammonia, drain cleaners, strong caustic solutions for cleaning reusable filters, and oven cleaners.
- Disposable masks for persons sensitive to powdered soap or detergent dust.
- Hair nets in food preparation and serving areas to minimize contamination of food.

Housekeeping

- Heavy rubber aprons and impervious gloves for persons engaged primarily in removal of nonhazardous trash.
- Protective gloves for users of soaps, detergents, or solvents.
- Appropriate gloves and face/eye protection when handling hazardous or infectious waste. The Material Safety Data Sheet (MSDS) for the hazardous chemical being handled will specify appropriate personal protective equipment.
- Nonskid shoes or boots for persons who flush, strip, rinse, and wax floors.

Laboratories

- Chemical goggles or face shields for protection from splashes.
- Chemical-cartridge respirators for persons cleaning up spills or using large amounts of acid, bases, and so forth.
- Coats or aprons, which are removed when wearers leave the laboratory.
- All other personal protective equipment specified in MSDSs or required for protection from infection, such as appropriate gloves or a face mask or apron.

Laundry

- Protective clothing and masks for sorting contaminated linen.
- Appropriate gloves for handling potentially infectious linen.
- Gloves, aprons, and safety glasses for persons using bleaches and soaps.
- Hair nets to minimize contamination of clean linen.

There are many additional health hazards commonly found in maintenance areas. These include:

- Asbestos often was used as an insulating material for steam pipes in older buildings.
- Carbon monoxide is given off by gasoline-powered engines on auxiliary power generators.
- Drain-cleaning chemicals can damage the eyes and burn the skin.
- Noise exposure exceeding allowable limits often occurs in boiler rooms.
- Paints and adhesives contain a wide variety of solvents. These compounds should only be used in areas that are adequately ventilated.
- Pesticides are used throughout the facility for fumigation and extermination of pests.
- Welding fumes expose employees to the fumes of the metals being joined and the filler material used. Excessive exposures can occur when maintenance personnel weld in confined spaces or other areas that do not have adequate ventilation and/or fume evacuation ducts.

Central Supply

Receiving, packaging, processing, and distribution operations occur in central supply. The major responsibility of the department focuses on materials handling. The following safety and health concerns are common in central supply:

- Cuts, bruises, and puncture wounds from blades, needles, knives, and broken glass often occur. Employees should handle returned items based on the assumption that they contain sharp or hazardous instruments and should be dealt with in accordance with universal blood and body fluid precautions.
- Strains, sprains, and back injuries also frequently occur in central supply areas. Therefore, employees should be instructed in proper materials-handling techniques.
- Sterilization equipment must be used properly to prevent burns from steam and overexposure to ethylene oxide (EtO). Employers must be in compliance with OSHA's EtO Standard (29 CFR 1910.1047). Compliance with this standard includes employee training, monitoring, medical surveillance, and the use of protective equipment.
- Chairs, boxes, and other objects inappropriately used for climbing are common causes of falls. Step stools and stepladders should be available to employees who need to reach high shelves in storage areas.
- Care must be taken to avoid damaging cylinders during handling and storage. (See the section on Compressed Gas Safety Program on p. 36.)

☐ Related Safety Considerations

Two other areas related to support service that require safety programs should be considered. These are construction safety and helicopter safety.

Construction and Renovation Safety

It is important that construction areas within and around the health care facility be safe not only for the construction workers but also for the health care community. A number of agencies, including OSHA and the Environmental Protection Agency (EPA), set safety standards for construction or renovation projects. During these projects, it is the responsibility of the construction managers and the facility engineering departments to enforce these standards.

The JCAHO requires Interim Life Safety Measures (ILSM), which are a series of 11 administrative actions that must be taken to temporarily compensate for the hazards posed by existing Life Safety Code deficiencies or construction activities. To ensure employee and patient safety during construction, the facility should follow certain guidelines. These include:

- Exits must allow people to leave freely without encountering obstructions. Personnel must receive training if alternative exits are designated.
- Free and unobstructed access must be provided to emergency departments or services and for emergency forces.
- Additional firefighting equipment must be provided and personnel trained in its use.
- Smoking must be prohibited in, or adjacent to, all construction areas.
- Storage, housekeeping, and debris-removal policies and procedures must be developed and enforced that reduce the flammable and combustible fire load to the lowest level necessary for daily operations.
- Hazard surveillance of buildings, grounds, and equipment must be increased with special attention to excavations, construction areas, construction storage, and field offices.

Helicopter Safety

To set up a helicopter program, the facility should research the services available in the area and the safety records of the organizations offering such services. The American Society of Hospital-Based Emergency Air Medical Services (ASHBEAMS) sets standards for the quality of patient care and the safety of operation of its more than 150 member programs. ASHBEAMS can provide information on the availability and quality of helicopter programs in the facility's area. Additionally, when the facility establishes or contracts with an air medical transport service, it must develop policies and procedures to protect the safety of patients and ground personnel.

Once the services of a medical air transport company have been contracted, the facility must prepare a landing pad that meets Federal Aviation Authority (FAA) requirements. The authority having jurisdiction over the landing and use of medical air transport, which may be the fire or police department or another department, should be contacted for restrictions on the location of this site. A rooftop landing pad may not always be the best choice because of the difficulties it may present for fire, police, or other personnel to reach the pad if they need to become involved.

During a disaster or other emergency, or if a regular landing pad is not established, it may be necessary to set up a field landing site. A plan should address what type of place will be used in this situation; a playground, open field, or parking lot is best. Personnel involved in this landing must have expertise in medical air evacuation and helicopter site procedures. Many factors such as mountainous or rough terrain, winds, bodies of water, and thermal currents can affect the size and type of landing zone required.

The field site should meet basic FAA safety requirements. When a helicopter has been called to an emergency field site, all major obstructions should be removed and flares should be set up to mark the zone. Lights or flares also should designate the presence of poles, wires, power lines, or signs that the pilot may have difficulty seeing.

□ Personal Protective Equipment

Recommendations were made in the preceding sections for protecting employees against specific departmental health care hazards. In addition to the protective equipment recommendations made, other types of protective clothing and equipment must be worn to protect against more general safety hazards. Examples of personal protective equipment include:

- Eye protection
- Foot protection
- Hand protection
- Body and face protection
- Ear protection
- Head protection

Eye Protection

Eye protection includes goggles, splash shields, welding glasses or hoods, and laser glasses. This equipment protects the eyes from chemical splashes, dust particles, body fluids, or hot sparks. Equipment should be selected to provide maximum protection for the intended application, and should be easy to clean and disinfect.

Foot Protection

Safety shoes are recommended to prevent injury to the feet from falling objects and other hazards. Safety shoes are particularly important where heavy materials are handled, such as in shipping and receiving operations. The engineering department may require its employees to wear steel-toe shoes to prevent injury from equipment and machinery.

Hand Protection

Hand protection generally is achieved by wearing gloves, and a wide variety of gloves utilized by health care facilities are available on the market. Gloves protect against cuts, abrasions, chemicals, heat, cold, and contamination by body fluids.

However, not all gloves offer the same protection. This is especially true in the case of handling liquids such as chemicals, blood, or body fluids, because some gloves do not provide a barrier to certain liquids. Thus, it is important to use gloves appropriate to the particular job. For example, laboratory and medical personnel wear gloves that protect their hands from contact with blood and body fluids, whereas engineering department employees wear a spark- or fire-retardant glove for handling welding equipment and a softer glove for moving equipment and for construction work.

It is equally important to ensure that gloves are not damaged. Damaged or worn gloves should be replaced.

Body and Face Protection

Body and face protection is achieved through clothing that includes items such as coveralls, masks, gowns, and aprons. As is the case with gloves, appropriate protective clothing is available for the performance of certain tasks. For example, disposable jumpsuits are worn by maintenance personnel to work on equipment in the sterile or surgical areas of the facility; surgical scrubs are worn by medical personnel to protect patients and to maintain a sterile environment in high-risk areas of the facility; and lab coats are worn by lab personnel to protect personal clothing from blood and chemical splashes.

Ear Protection

Damaged ears or hearing loss can be avoided by wearing the proper hearing protection—for example, earplugs or earmuffs. In addition, steps can be taken to alter the environment. For example, sometimes the length of exposure to loud noises can be shortened or the level of noise can be reduced by redesigning or enclosing machinery. Employees must use hearing protection in areas of extreme noise such as construction areas and during helicopter landings.

Many different kinds of hearing protectors are available. Choosing the right one for each individual depends on several factors, including the following:

- The amount of protection needed
- Comfort
- Fit with other equipment being worn, such as head and eye protection

Special caution needs to be taken with hearing protectors. Earplugs should be kept clean by washing them with soap and water, and should not be shared because ear infections can be contagious. Disposable earplugs should be thrown away and damaged earmuffs replaced.

Head Protection

Head protection is achieved principally by wearing headgear such as a hard hat. Hard hats are designed to absorb blows to the head and usually are required in construction areas. They help prevent serious injury in the following ways:

- The hard shell resists and deflects the blow, distributing the impact over a larger area. The hat suspension acts as a shock absorber. Even if the hat dents or shatters, it still takes some force out of the blow.
- Some hats are modified to shield the scalp, face, neck, and shoulders against splashes or spills.
- Some hard hats allow the addition of other protection such as goggles, hearing protection, face shields, and hoods.

The hard hat should fit properly and should not be left out in the sun, because sunlight and heat can deteriorate the shell. When a hat is cracked or has received a serious blow, it should be discarded.

☐ Safety Considerations for All Health Care Workers

In addition to on-site staff, the health care facility also must consider the safety needs of two other groups who often are exposed to safety hazards. These groups are volunteers and hospital-based home health service employees.

Volunteers

Because volunteers often are involved in activities that take them into virtually all areas of the facility, management and administration should take special care to see that they are protected. Volunteers will need safety training for tasks they perform, such as moving patients in wheelchairs or stretchers, lifting or moving boxes and equipment, and providing clerical support services. In addition, volunteers should participate in fire and disaster preparedness training to assist in the event of an emergency. They also should wear identification badges and appropriate clothing such as nonskid shoes.

Home Health Service Employees

Although hospital-based home care staff are exposed to many of the same hazards as employees who work in hospitals, home environments may provide many more opportunities for injury because homes are not designed to industrial safety standards. In addition, housekeeping standards and practices may be below those required for maximum safety. Hazards to which home health employees are exposed include the following:

- Viruses such as TB, HBV, and HIV
- Hazardous chemicals
- Infectious materials and waste
- Compressed gases, including handling and storage of medical gas cylinders
- Strains, sprains, and back injuries from handling equipment and patients
- Injuries from handling sharps
- Violent patient behavior
- Fire and other emergencies, such as the use of oxygen and smoking in bed
- Inadequate electrical wiring
- Storage and handling of drugs
- Slippery surfaces
- Tripping hazards, such as throw rugs and improperly stored material

In order to ensure staff and patient safety and health during home health care, governmental regulations and the JCAHO require that employees must be trained according to the same standards required of health care facilities. Examples of training that must be provided include the following:

- Information about the requirements of the OSHA Hazard Communication Standard
- Information on employer and employee rights and responsibilities under the Hazard Communication Standard
- How to determine potentially hazardous chemicals
- Information on how to protect themselves from work environment hazards, including the use of personal protective equipment and proper work practices
- Infection control precautions, including bloodborne pathogens, TB, and hazardous waste disposal
- Safe and appropriate use of medical equipment
- Storage and handling of medical gases and drugs
- Procedures for reporting, documenting, and investigating accidents, injuries, and safety hazards

- Use of equipment to ensure it is used in a safe manner and is working as intended
- Fire response, use of smoke detectors, hazards of smoking in bed, and procedures for summoning emergency assistance
- Electrical safety, including proper use of extension cords, plugs, space heaters, and heating pads
- Environmental and mobility safety, such as the use of throw rugs, stair climbing, furniture arrangement, floor surfaces, and proper lighting
- Bathroom safety, including the use of grab bars and bath benches
- Medication safety
- Employee personal safety in neighborhoods visited
- Defensive driving

☐ Conclusion

To ensure safe and healthful working conditions in the health care facility, it is essential that departmental safety practices be implemented in addition to the facilitywide safety program. These practices must be designed to address safety hazards that are unique to each department within both the clinical care areas and support services. Guidelines should include not only steps to be taken to avoid safety hazards but also the personal protective equipment that employees should wear when exposed to each hazard. Additionally, the facility should ensure that those guidelines apply to personnel such as volunteers and hospital-based home service employees.

Once departmental safety guidelines have been described in specific policies and procedures, they should be reviewed and updated regularly. They should then fit into the facility's comprehensive safety management program as part of the hospital's systematic approach to safety.

Patient Safety

During patient care, many accidents and injuries can occur. Several factors conspire to jeopardize patient safety, including effects of medication, weakness from surgery, or general agitation resulting from illness. Patients may overestimate their ability to stand, walk, or perform other normal routine activities. Or, they may be dissatisfied with their care and treatment and lash out at facility personnel. Some elderly patients suffering from Alzheimer's disease or senility may become agitated and abuse staff, family, or visitors.

These conditions and others may predispose patients to injuries sustained through slips, falls, and burns. Patient care procedures such as lifting and transporting from one area of the facility to another also may cause injury, especially to the fragile bones of elderly patients. Additionally, all of these incidents constitute potentially compensable events for which patients may file claims and recover damages.

Employee and patient safety converge in nearly every patient care activity, as well as in many tasks not directly related to patient care. For example, during patient lifting, not only could the patient fall or twist a limb but the caregiver doing the lifting also could experience strain or sprain to the back or muscles. And unmarked wet floors could cause patient, employee, volunteer, or visitor to fall. Through attention to patient safety, the facility will (1) reduce accidents and potentially compensable events among both employees and patients, (2) enhance overall safety in the facility, and (3) improve patient care.

This chapter presents some of the principal safety issues concerning patients in the health care facility. It also considers the safety of patients with special needs and the importance of establishing good patient relations.

□ Common Considerations in Patient Safety

Certain circumstances commonly present the potential for patient injury in the health care facility. The following subsections describe these circumstances and the dangers they can pose to both patients and health care workers.

Lifting and Transporting Patients

By most measures, back injuries and muscle strain from lifting patients represent the single greatest class of injury to health care workers, especially nurses, orderlies, and nurses' aides. These injuries can occur when health care personnel help patients to stand, transfer patients to chairs or wheelchairs, or move patients to gurneys. Moreover, patients also run the risk of being severely injured in lifting accidents.

Despite the apparent difficulty of the task, the safe lifting of patients is possible. In fact, most injuries result from improper lifting techniques. It is essential that all personnel involved in lifting patients be trained in lifting techniques. Some institutions restrict lifts and transfers to trained lifting teams. Employee back injuries and patient fractures and contusions can be very serious, leading to pain, liability, and costly workers' compensation claims. Providing adequate training and implementing safe practices can minimize this major risk to employees, patients, and the facility. The plan of care should identify the safest method of transfer for both patient and caregiver. The plan also should specify that a physical therapy consultation be carried out for difficult transfer patients.

When transferring patients to a chair or wheelchair, a sequence of steps should be followed. The health care worker should:

1. Sum up the situation and plan the lift.
2. Ask for help when necessary. A patient weight and mobility policy should be established that mandates getting help or using a mechanical device before the patient is lifted.
3. Explain to the patient what is going to take place prior to the move.
4. Position the chair or wheelchair parallel to the bed and lock both bed casters and wheelchair wheels. The bed should be adjusted to the correct height to facilitate the transfer.
5. Loosen the bedclothes for easier motion.
6. Slide the patient into position, by pushing or pulling.
7. Ask the patient to assist in flexing the knees, if possible.
8. Place one arm under the patient's knees and the other under his or her far shoulder.
9. Help the patient to a seated position with his or her feet on the floor.
10. Stand with feet slightly apart for good balance, bending at the knees and hips.
11. Ask the patient to clasp arms around the worker's neck, if possible.
12. Hold the patient close, straightening legs to lift and pushing with thigh muscles.
13. Shift foot position to turn. The torso should not be twisted.
14. Maintain a firm but gentle hold on the patient, while completing the transfer.

The first nine steps also can be used to help a patient sit up in bed. However, instead of allowing the patient's feet to hang over the edge, the patient's upper body should be moved to a vertical position against the headboard, with his or her legs extended on the bed.

In most cases in which a patient's entire body must be lifted, three people should participate. One person supports the patient's head and shoulders, one supports the midsection, and one holds the legs. They then roll the patient onto his or her side so that their arms cradle the section each holds. They lift and turn to place the patient on the gurney or stretcher.

Some lifting aids are available, such as draw sheets and mechanical lifting devices. In using a draw sheet, one person stands on either side of the patient. The sheet is held at the patient's shoulders and buttocks, pulled tight, and the patient is moved across the bed.

Mechanical lifting devices may be used in lifting particularly large or unresponsive patients. However, employees must be trained in the safe use of such devices and their limitations. The manufacturer's instructions must always be followed.

By practicing the proper lifting and transporting techniques, health care workers will ensure not only their safety but also the safety of their patients.

Preventing Slips and Falls

Studies consistently show that falls represent the single greatest cause of injury to patients. Although risk factors may differ widely from facility to facility, the one that is most often associated with frequent falls is age. Patients over 65 are more likely to fall and to suffer more serious injuries, such as hip and limb fractures. Hip fractures can so disable an elderly individual that he or she must be placed in a nursing home. Other patient groups at greater risk of slips and falls are the mentally disturbed, those with weakened physical conditions, and those taking psychoactive drugs or a combination of medications.

Research also indicates that the great majority of falls occur in patient rooms, most within a few feet of the bed or en route to the private bathroom. However, falls are in no way limited to these areas or to patients. Elderly visitors also run the risk of falling in hallways and patient rooms. Every facility must assess which patients are at risk and take preventive measures.

By far, the single most effective preventive measure is basic housekeeping. It is the responsibility of each employee to make sure patients are not exposed to slip and fall hazards. Spills of liquids such as water, food, and urine are frequent causes of falls. If a spill cannot be cleaned up immediately, a safety cone should be used to warn of a slipping hazard. Spills also can be prevented by delivering liquids in spill-proof containers or on trays, rather than in individual pitchers or containers that will spill if dropped on the floor.

Storage of equipment, boxes, and other items on the floor or in the corridor also endangers patient safety. If equipment must be stored in the corridor temporarily, it should be kept to one side and extend into the corridor no further than 24 inches. It must not block patient room or fire doors.

Some facilities have instituted programs to identify fall-prone patients at admittance. Several factors can be assessed to determine degree of risk. For example:

- History of having fallen at home
- Poor eyesight
- Unsteady gait
- Combination of prescriptions
- Preoperative or postoperative conditions
- Uncooperative or belligerent attitude

Hospital staff should take action to reduce the risk of falls for all patients. By identifying fall-prone patients at time of admission, staff can focus attention on eliminating all risks pertinent to this type of patient. For example, the number of times a fall-prone patient goes to the bathroom during the night can be reduced by taking the patient to the bathroom before he or she goes to sleep for the night. Additionally, identification of fall-prone patients allows staff to be particularly watchful during busy morning hours when such patients normally go to the bathroom. Fall-prone patients can be identified through some visible means of identification, such as red tape on their ID bracelets or kardex. The kardex list is updated throughout the day. (See figure 5-1 for a sample daily fall-prevention list.)

In addition to a formal program of patient fall prevention, caregivers should know at least certain basic fall-prevention measures. For example:

- Patient belongings and call buttons should be kept close to the bed so that patients do not have to reach too far for them, thus avoiding slipping and falling. Similarly, call buttons should be placed within reach in the bathroom, close to the commode and shower.
- Patients should be educated with fall-prevention programs.
- Lighting in corridors and public areas should be kept bright.
- Patients should be encouraged to go to the bathroom before they go to sleep at night. This simple measure can help reduce nighttime falls.
- Any medication that contributes to frequent falls and disorientation should be reevaluated.
- Nursing home residents should be helped to correct physical disabilities through physical therapy and walking aids.
- Nursing coverage should be increased during high-risk activities, such as getting out of bed and going to the bathroom.
- Hostile patients should be subdued. Anger and resentment have been shown to contribute to falls.
- Softer surfaces for floors or furniture should be introduced, and grab bars and handrails provided throughout the facility.
- Safety devices such as nonslip surfaces and footstools with rubber feet should be used.
- Bed rails should be used.

Figure 5-1.   Daily Patient Fall Prevention List

Date: _____   Unit: _____

Date Listed	Time Listed	Name	Age	Room Number	Listed	RN Initials

Comments: _____

_____

[The following is] to be completed by Head Nurse or designated RN at end of 24-hour period.

Total Number of Patient Falls	Number of Falls by Patients Listed	Number of Falls by Patients Not Listed	Number of Incident Reports	Signature of Head Nurse or Designated RN

Reprinted, with permission, from Wade, R. D. *Risk Management—HPL, Hospital Professional Liability Primer.* Columbus, OH: Ohio Hospital Insurance Co., 1981.

- Torn carpeting should be repaired and other obstructions removed from patient areas.
- The patient's personal footwear, such as slippers and shoes, should be inspected and replaced if slippery.

Through staff involvement and a philosophy of prevention, the facility can significantly reduce dangerous and costly patient falls.

Preventing Burns

Another common cause of patient injury is burns, and a common source of patient burns is hot food spills. Because they are unaccustomed to eating in bed, patients may easily spill hot coffee, tea, and soups. Nurses should be aware of patients such as children and the elderly who may be likely to spill hot foods or liquids. These patients should be supervised while they eat, and assistance should be provided if necessary.

Another possible source of burns is prescribed heat treatments, such as heating pads or steam inhalators. Patients undergoing heat treatments must be carefully monitored to ensure that they can tolerate them. Oxygen-enriched atmospheres, accompanied by a spark or other heat source, can set patient clothing and bedding on fire, resulting in patient burns and room fires.

Many electrical appliances and outlets within the facility create the potential for shocks and burns. (See figure 5-2 for a summary of safety tips to prevent injuries from these devices.) In addition to ensuring their safe operation, the facility should discourage patients from bringing personal electrical devices from home. If a patient does bring an electrical device to the facility, the biomedical or engineering department should do an electrical safety check on the equipment and check the electrical load requirements before the equipment is used. Although the facility is still liable if the patient is electrocuted, a well-written and documented electrical safety check program will go far in providing proof that the facility tried to prevent patient injury.

Enforcing Patient Smoking Guidelines

To provide a more healthful environment and to reduce the risk of fire, many health care organizations have established a smoke-free environment throughout their facilities. Nevertheless, in those areas where smoking is not prohibited, the facility must develop, implement, and enforce strict patient smoking guidelines which every patient should know and understand. For example, smoking should never be permitted in areas where oxygen is in use because of the risk of fire. In addition, patient conditions such as disorientation, certain psychiatric problems, senility, or suicidal tendencies may warrant severe restrictions on smoking privileges, such as allowing these patients to smoke only under close supervision.

Figure 5-2. Electrical Appliance Safety Measures

Heating pads and hot-water bottles

- Never place a heating pad or hot-water bottle directly against an unconscious person, a person in shock, an infant, or a dressing.
- Check the temperature of pads and bottles. Temperatures should never exceed 130° F (54.4° C) for adults and 120° F (48.8° C) for children.
- Check skin temperature shortly after applying a pad or bottle. Do not accept the patient's opinion on his or her comfort.
- Check soundness of each item before use. Heating pads are electrical appliances and subject to all regulations set for electrical equipment.
- Use tape, binders, or straps to keep units in place. Do not use pins or clamps.
- Use heating pad only on low setting.

Infrared lamps and light cradles

- Use infrared lamps and light cradles only on the physician's orders.
- If the site to be treated is near the head, protect the patient's eyes with a towel or washcloth.
- Place the equipment at least 18 inches from the patient's body. In a light cradle only a 25-watt bulb is used.
- Ensure that equipment has guards.
- Attend the patient the entire time the equipment is in use. The attendant must be a staff member, not a visitor.
- Inspect wiring and connections daily.

Steam inhalators

- Inspect the steam inhalator equipment before using it to be sure it is filled with water.
- Prevent hot vapor from concentrating on the patient's body.
- Make sure the equipment does not overheat.
- Do not place steam inhalators on bedside tables where patients may accidentally knock them over.

All burns require immediate attention and notification of the patient's physician.

Personal electrical appliances

- Use of personal electrical appliances should be limited.
- Elderly persons, children, and patients with psychiatric conditions should be closely supervised while using personal electrical appliances.
- Check these appliances when they are brought in and, for long-term care residents, regularly thereafter for worn wiring, connections, and plugs.

Additionally, nonsmoking patients should be given the right to protest being placed in the same room with a smoker. Sensitive situations can be handled delicately by quickly responding to the request before animosity develops.

Minimizing Medication Errors

Among the other common and potentially very serious accidents in health care facilities are medication errors. To minimize medication errors, the responsibilities of all those involved in the prescribing, filling, and administering of medication should be adequately defined. Those health care personnel involved include the attending physician and the pharmacist, as well as the attending nurse. Some facilities use computerized dispensing of medications to reduce errors. In any case, errors can be avoided through good training and strict attention to detail.

The attending physician must issue written medication orders. Verbal orders must be countersigned by the physician within 48 hours. All orders must be legible, clear, and concise; and must include the patient's full name, the dosage, the time and duration of the prescription, and the name of the drug. The physician has responsibility for ensuring that others fully understand the order and for clarifying any ambiguity.

The pharmacist has responsibility for preparing and dispensing all medications exactly according to the prescribing physician's orders. The pharmacist should always contact the physician when orders are unclear, rather than guess at them. He or she must keep accurate records of the supplies of drugs and report any irregularities.

The attending nurse has responsibility for administering medications, except when the physician is legally the only one allowed to administer the drug. To prevent medication errors at this stage, the nurse should first realize that accurate drug administration requires a careful procedure that must be done slowly and deliberately. Rushing is a frequent contributor to medication errors. To reduce errors, a strict system of drug administration is required.

The process for administering medication involves a number of steps. These include:

1. All prescriptions should be checked in the order book to ensure that there are orders for the medication and that they have not changed.
2. Drugs should be kept in their original containers and labels should be checked to ensure that they are intact.
3. Medication should be returned to the pharmacy if it does not contain the following information:
   - Prescription number
   - Drug name
   - Drug strength
   - Name of the patient, physician, and pharmacy
   - Directions for use
   - Date of issue
4. All medications should be correctly identified under good light before they are measured.
5. The label should be read at least three times:
   - When removing the container from the storage cabinet
   - Before measuring the medication
   - When replacing the container in the storage cabinet
6. All medications should be carefully measured when they are not dispensed by unit doses in the pharmacy.
7. The prescribing physician should be contacted before the drug is administered if it is suspected that the patient's drug combination may have dangerous interactions.
8. The required time schedule for the administration of all pharmaceuticals should be strictly followed.
9. Patients should be identified in at least two ways before they are given medication. For example, the caregiver should ask their names and receive a positive response if they are alert, and then double-check by looking at their arm bands and charts.

10. The caregiver should stay with the patient until all the medicine has been consumed.
11. The caregiver should be alert to special precautions for the preparation, administration, and disposal of hazardous drugs, such as those used in cytotoxic and chemotherapy procedures.

It is essential that nurses be trained in this procedure and that the physician and the pharmacist be aware of their equal responsibility in minimizing medication errors.

All medication errors should be documented on an incident report. The safety committee should review medication errors regularly for trends or other problems, and then recommend and monitor corrective action. Consistent monitoring and ongoing staff education are important tools in reducing the potential for medication errors.

Using Restraints

During their stay at a health care facility, sometimes patients may need to be restrained to prevent them from causing injury to themselves or others. Restraining a patient may be one of the most difficult decisions that a health care provider has to make. Although the restraint may seem inhumane, the alternative of allowing patients to injure themselves or others may create far more serious problems.

One way to alleviate this source of concern is to train patient care staff and others involved with patient care in ways to discourage aggression. They should talk in a soothing manner and ask about the problem without appearing confrontational. Frequently, patients may be confused and apprehensive and their personalities may be altered by medication or other treatment. Understanding and empathy with the patient's position will help staff realize that the patient's aggressive behavior is not a personal attack. Employees should understand that good patient relations can minimize the likelihood of aggressive behavior.

However, invariably some patients will require restraint. In addition to using them with combative patients, restraints may be needed for senile patients and those under the influence of medication or alcohol. The decision to restrain should always be in response to a specific event that demonstrates the danger the patient presents. Restraints should never be used simply to prevent or punish violent behavior or just because patients sometimes show signs of dementia or aggression. An exception to this would be the patient who has a consistent record of sudden violence or of falls from beds or wheelchairs. If all other efforts to correct this condition have failed, the regular use of soft restraints is acceptable. The facility should be prepared to demonstrate a compelling reason for the use of restraints and all proper authorization should be obtained.

In the event that restraints are required, the safety of employees and other caregivers is as important as that of the patient. Employees who are required to restrain a patient must be thoroughly trained in the safety measures needed to avoid injury to themselves. The facility should implement a policy and procedure that specifies when restraint is appropriate, who should approve the decision, how the patient should be restrained, the maximum time the patient should be restrained, where the patient will be restrained, and the frequency of checks. The procedure on restraints should include the following elements:

- Restraints should be used if there is a clear and present danger to the patient, other patients, or staff. The provoking event should be documented in the patient's chart.
- The patient should be removed from populated areas before being restrained.
- The caregiver should explain to the patient what is being done and why. When possible, open discussion should be encouraged.
- The patient should be searched for matches or cigarettes before being restrained. He or she could use these items to get free of the restraints by burning them off.
- The caregiver should never restrain an unwilling patient alone.
- Either the attending physician or the physician on call should countersign the order to restrain.

- Only padded bed restraints should be used.
- The patient should be checked regularly for discomfort, chafing, tearing of fragile skin of the elderly, tightness, and so on. The checks should be documented in the chart.
- The caregiver should ensure that the restraints do not choke, scratch, or limit circulation.
- The prescribed time limits for physical restraint should never be exceeded.

When restraints are used, those involved must complete an incident report describing what happened and the restraining measures that were used. The documentation must adequately explain that efforts were made to subdue the patient, authorization was obtained, and regular checks were made. This report can serve as protection against liability, as a guide for investigating the event, or for reference at a later time should the event recur. (See figure 5-3 for a four-step approach to patient restraint.)

Using Call Systems

A call system acts as a tool for patient safety, but too often becomes a source of irritation and tension between nurse and patient. Nurses should recognize that call systems are designed to prevent patients from taking potentially dangerous steps to seek help—for example, climbing over bed rails or grabbing for an item out of reach.

To avoid misuse of the call system, nurses should explain to patients what they can and cannot do without assistance, and should show patients, family members, and visitors alike how to use the system. Patients and their families need to know the purpose of each button and any special features. Once the function of the system is understood, prompt and courteous responses to calls will encourage patients to use it.

Call buttons should be placed within patient reach. Some facilities attach the button to the patient's pillow, taking care that he or she cannot become entangled in the cord. In other

Figure 5-3. A Four-Step Approach to Restraint

1. Evaluate

- What characteristics is the patient displaying? Violent behavior? Falls from the bed or wheelchair? Self-destructiveness?
- Has the patient acted this way in the past?
- Does the patient's current behavior match predetermined criteria for restraint?
- Are there indications that the patient may resist restraint?
- Might it be possible to defuse the situation so that restraint is unnecessary?

2. Plan

- How quickly must the patient be restrained?
- How and with what is the patient to be restrained?
- Do we have the staff and equipment assembled before implementation?
- Do all the team members know the plan of action?

3. Implement

- Explain to the patient what will be done.
- Work together as a team.
- Minimize the audience. If possible, move the patient to a less public area before restraining.
- Treat the patient with dignity and respect.
- After restraining the patient, explain to him or her the reasons for the restraints and when they will be removed. Check the restraints and the patient frequently.

4. Document

- Detail in an incident report what occurred, what restraining measures were used, and the authorization received.
- Chart the incident, including the times the restrained patient was checked.
- Regularly review restraining incidents and learn from mistakes.

facilities, call buttons are located in bedside rails. Ensuring that call buttons are within patient reach prevents a major falling hazard that could result when patients attempt to use a button that is out of reach.

Some systems initiate an emergency call when a wall plug is pulled out. This action alarms a second location, such as the station of the facility telephone operator, as well as the nursing station. This type of system is valuable for responding to critically ill patients should the nursing station be temporarily unstaffed.

☐ Patients Requiring Special Considerations

Certain groups of patients have special needs and thus require special considerations on the part of facility staff. Among these diverse groups are elderly patients, pediatric patients, and culturally diverse patients.

Elderly Patients

The fastest-growing age group in America today is composed of individuals over age 65. In what has been called the "graying of America," people are living longer than ever before and in larger numbers. This trend can be expected to continue as the baby boomers reach middle and old age, and has a great bearing on health care. Older people can experience a greater number of health problems than their younger counterparts.

Although many of these patients will be in surprisingly good mental and physical condition, the greater number of senior citizens increases the likelihood that facilities will encounter more patients who are senile, physically disabled, and often depressed. In elderly patients, vision often is not good; anxiety and isolation may cause disorientation or contribute to senility; balance may be delicate; and poor circulation may make patients prone to dizziness. In addition, sometimes elderly patients are incontinent, which presents safety issues as well as issues associated with maintaining patient dignity; and many patients take drugs that may make them more susceptible to a variety of accidents. It also is common for the elderly to have fragile skin, which requires that they be handled with a light touch.

Because of these special problems, many facilities have set up programs to educate staff about the needs of elderly patients in an effort to promote understanding and compassion. The facility may have someone knowledgeable about aging discuss its effects and the ways personnel can alleviate problems. For example, shadows may confuse elderly patients, causing them to misjudge a step and fall. Further, there have been instances in which confused elderly patients have wandered away from the facility and have been hit by an automobile or died from exposure. In addition, abuse and neglect are more common with elderly patients, whose unresponsiveness or disabilities may frustrate staff members. A comprehensive staff education program can help prevent such incidents.

In addition to general training and education, nursing home staff and hospital personnel who care for the elderly should be trained specifically in geriatric care. Treatment and care of the elderly can differ greatly from acute care for younger patients. Besides safety and liability prevention, staff trained in geriatrics will be better equipped to deal with the deep emotional concerns and unique health conditions of older patients. This training will appreciably affect the quality of care the facility offers to this burgeoning sector of the population.

Pediatric Patients

Pediatric patients also present unique risks, especially when they are young and mobile. For example, they may stray from their room or even from the floor and become lost or suffer injury. Additionally, young surgery patients may injure themselves if they become too rambunctious. Their use of bed rails, wheelchairs, and so on for fun may cause accidents. In recent years in particular, kidnapping and estranged parents have become a primary concern.

Although family members often spend a great deal of time with pediatric patients, the facility is still responsible for their safety and must not relinquish that responsibility to the family. Training and procedures need to be developed to ensure that staff can handle the responsibility and safety of pediatric patients.

Culturally Diverse Patients

The most common cultural difference between patients and caregivers is language. Differences in language can create safety problems resulting from poor understanding and inadequate communication. Many individuals from different ethnic backgrounds understand less English than is apparent by their conversation. Staff should be aware of the potential for misunderstanding and use special care when giving instructions or listening to patient requests. Ways to help ensure that patients understand important information about their care include using an interpreter, using international sign language, or asking patients for feedback on what they have been told. If indications are that communication is not good, staff should follow up on critical instructions to ensure that they are being followed.

Other diversity differences relate to the variety of personal needs that affect patient comfort and attitude. Diversity occurs because of differences in sex, ethnic and/or religious background, and personality traits (such as modesty and temperament). Following are some of the special considerations that patients with diversity differences may require:

- Diets to meet religious needs—for example, kosher or vegetarian meals
- Covering and bed baths by staff of the same sex for self-conscious patients
- Room temperature and the amount of bedclothes
- Sensitivity to noise and light
- Anxiety about procedures or shots that may affect the patient's ability to rest

☐ Conclusion

Patient safety should be at the heart of the health care facility's safety program. The patient has come to the facility with the hope not only of being healed but also of staying in a safe environment and being treated kindly and with respect. In setting out to deliver health care, the facility has made a commitment to serve its community through high-quality patient care. The facility must preserve patient safety through protection from accidents resulting from improper use of restraints, unsuccessful lifting techniques, slips, falls, burns, and medication errors. Instead of just following checklists for basic safety, the facility must incorporate a philosophy that emphasizes the importance of safety and compassion in patient treatment. Only through integrating these elements into a system of total care can the facility fulfill its obligation to serve the community.

Hazardous Materials Management

C hemicals and drugs make our lives easier in many ways. However, these materials that are so beneficial also can be hazardous and can complicate our lives with risks of damage to health or the environment.

Health care facilities handle and store a wide variety of hazardous materials throughout their facilities. Protecting employees from exposure to these materials requires an integrated hazardous materials management program. This program involves training employees in safe handling techniques and developing methods for handling, storing, and disposing of hazardous materials prior to bringing them into the facility.

Depending on the facility, the hazardous materials management program may be the responsibility of an individual specifically chosen for this task or it may be incorporated in the facilitywide safety program. This chapter provides a broad overview of the various hazardous materials programs that must be in place in order to meet regulatory requirements and to provide a safe and healthy work environment.

□ Hazard Communication Standard

A comprehensive hazardous materials management plan begins before the chemicals arrive at the facility. It requires that staff members record what chemicals are being used in each department, their hazards, and other pertinent information. (See figure 6-1 for a list of common hazardous materials and where they may be found in the health care facility.) It also mandates that employees be trained in the proper ways to handle the hazardous materials in order to reduce risks to their safety and health.

In the mid-1970s, the Occupational Safety and Health Administration (OSHA) noticed that growing numbers of employees were working with chemicals without knowing the hazards involved and were thus unable to protect themselves. In many cases, employers knew little or nothing about the chemicals. Alarmed at this situation, OSHA published the Hazard Communication Standard (OSHA 29 CFR 1910.1200). This standard proposed that workers have a "right to know" (see chapter 2) about the chemicals with which they work.

To ensure workers' right to know, the standard requires that employers take several specific actions. The major requirements are as follows:

- *Hazard determination:* This part of the Hazard Communication Standard pertains primarily to manufacturers and importers of hazardous chemicals. Hazard determination refers to extensive research that these businesses must conduct on the hazards of the chemicals they manufacture or sell. To maintain accuracy, businesses must review and update this research regularly. The results of the hazard determination are then used to write material safety data sheets for all the chemicals.

Figure 6-1. Areas of a Health Care Facility Where Hazardous Materials and Wastes May Be Found

- *Laboratory or Pathology:* formaldehyde, alcohol, acetone, acetylene, hydrogen gas, nitrogen gas, radioisotopes, hydrochloric acid, sulfuric acid, picric acid, sodium hydroxide, benzene, toluene, ammonium hydroxide, bleach, xylene, blood, blood products, sharps, bacteria, viruses, fungi, and body parts
- *Radiology:* alcohols, acetone, sharps, oxygen, acids, bases, and body fluids
- *Central Supply:* ethylene oxide, alcohols, acetone, bleach, phenols, acids, body fluids, and quartenary amines
- *Materials Management:* acids, bases, alcohols, toluene, xylene, solvents, gases, paints, thinners, degreasers, bleach, cleaners, phenols, and quartenary amines
- *Engineering or Plant Operations:* solvents, adhesives, adhesive removers, thinners, paints, lacquer, alcohols, acetone, toluene, acids, bases, phenols, quartenary amines, degreasers, welding rods, acetylene, oxygen, gasoline, and ethylene glycol
- *Dietary:* cleaners, degreasers, lye, bases, acids, phenols, quartenary amines, and methanol
- *Housekeeping:* acids, bases, aerosols, alcohols, methylene chloride, bleach, phenols, quartenary amines, polishes, strippers, and spot or stain removers
- *Groundskeeping:* pesticides, herbicides, gasoline, fertilizer, alcohol, acetone, toluene, xylene, paints, and ethylene glycol
- *Laundry:* bases, acids, bleach, methylene chloride, phenols, quartenary amines, oils, lubricants, and other disinfectants
- *Print Shop:* alcohols, caustics, corrosives, flammables, cleaners, degreasers, toluene, acetic acid, acetone, xylene, toner, and fixatives
- *Nuclear Medicine:* radionuclides, blood, other body fluids, alcohol, acetone, acids, bases, bleach, phenols, quartenary amines, and sharps
- *Oncology:* antineoplastic chemicals, alcohols, acetone, blood, body fluids, sharps, bleach, and other disinfectants
- *Pharmacy:* all types of antineoplastic chemicals, alcohols, acetones, solvents, acids, bases, phenols, quartenary amines, and bleach
- *Surgery:* ethylene oxide, anesthetic gases, alcohols, solvents, acetone, oxygen, other compressed gases, formaldehyde, phenols, bleach, quartenary amines, blood, sharps, and other body fluids
- *Emergency Department:* acids, bases, alcohols, acetones, solvents, bleach, phenols, quartenary amines, oxygen, anesthetic gases, other compressed gases, blood, sharps, and other body fluids

- *Material safety data sheets (MSDSs):* MSDSs are documents that provide detailed information on chemicals, including the hazards they present, personal protective equipment (PPE) to be used, and emergency procedures to be followed. (See figure 6-2 for a sample MSDS form.)
- *Container labeling:* Employers must ensure that all chemicals in the facility are labeled with the proper identification and health warnings. Although most chemicals arrive at the facility labeled, many of them often are repoured into containers not labeled for them. Thus, a procedure must be in place to ensure that all chemicals are properly labeled.
- *Hazardous chemical list:* Facilities must compile a list of all the hazardous chemicals they use or produce, and make this list available to employees.
- *Written hazard communication program:* The facility must explain in writing how it proposes to comply with OSHA's Hazard Communication regulations. The resulting document is a handbook titled *Hazard Communication Program,* which is used in the facility's program of compliance and training.
- *Employee information and training:* Employers must provide extensive information and training. Employees must be trained in:
  —The standard's requirements
  —The facility's written *Hazard Communication Program*
  —What chemicals they may be exposed to in their work
  —Where the MSDSs, lists of chemicals, and a copy of the written *Hazard Communication Program* are located
  —The hazards of the chemicals in their areas
  —How to recognize and handle the hazardous chemicals in their areas
  —The use of protective measures

Figure 6-2. Material Safety Data Sheet

Material Safety Data Sheet

QUICK IDENTIFIER
Common Name: (used on label and list)

May be used to comply with OSHA's Hazard Communication Standard,
29CFR 1910. 1200. Standard must be consulted for specific requirements.

SECTION 1 -

Manufacturer's
Name

Address

Emergency
Telephone No.

City, State, and ZIP

Other
Information
Calls

Signature of Person
Responsible for Preparation (Optional)

Date
Prepared

SECTION 2 – HAZARDOUS INGREDIENTS/IDENTITY

Hazardous Component(s) (chemical & common name(s))	OSHA PEL	ACGIH TLV	Other Exposure Limits	% (optional)	CAS NO.

SECTION 3 – PHYSICAL & CHEMICAL CHARACTERISTICS

Boiling Point	Specific Gravity (H₂O=1)	Vapor Pressure (mm Hg)

Vapor Density (Air = 1)

Solubility in Water — Reactivity in Water

Appearance and Odor — Melting Point

SECTION 4 – FIRE & EXPLOSION DATA

Flash Point F. C. Method Used — Flammable Limits in Air % by Volume LEL Lower UEL Upper

Auto-Ignition Temperature — Extinguisher Media

Special Fire Fighting Procedures

Unusual Fire and Explosion Hazards

Note: This is page 1 of a two-page form.

(Continued on next page)

Figure 6-2. (Continued)

SECTION 5 – PHYSICAL HAZARDS (REACTIVITY DATA)

Stability   Unstable ☐ Conditions
            Stable ☐   to Avoid

Incompatability
(Materials to Avoid)

Hazardous
Decomposition Products

Hazardous   May Occur ☐   Conditions
Polymerization Will Not Occur ☐ to Avoid

SECTION 6 – HEALTH HAZARDS

1. Acute   2. Chronic

Signs and
Symptoms of Exposure

Medical Conditions Generally
Aggravated by Exposure

Chemical Listed as Carcinogen or Potential Carcinogen	National Toxicology Program	Yes No	I.A.R.C. Monographs	Yes ☐ No ☐	OSHA	Yes ☐ No ☐

Emergency and
First Aid Procedures

ROUTES OF ENTRY
1. Inhalation
2. Eyes
3. Skin
4. Ingestion

SECTION 7 – SPECIAL PRECAUTIONS AND SPILL/LEAK PROCEDURES

Precautions to be Taken
in Handling and Storage

Other
Precautions

Steps to be Taken in Case
Material is Released or Spilled

Waste Disposal
Methods (Consult federal, state, and local regulations)

SECTION 8 – SPECIAL PROTECTION INFORMATION/CONTROL MEASURES

Respiratory Protection
(Specify Type)

Ventilation	Local Exhaust	Mechanical (General)	Special	Other

Protective   Eye
Gloves   Protection

Other Protective
Clothing or Equipment

Work/Hygienic Practices

IMPORTANT
Do not leave any blank spaces. If required information is unavailable, unknown, or does not apply, so indicate.

CU-F1R   Printed by Labelmaster, Division of American Labelmark Company, Inc.   Chicago, IL 60646-6719   1-800-621-5808 ● (321) 478-0900

- *Contractor procedure:* The facility must advise outside contractors of any chemical hazards they may encounter in the normal course of their work. In addition, each contractor who brings chemicals on-site must provide the facility with hazard information for these substances before the chemicals are brought into the facility.

OSHA has in place an inspection process to ensure facility compliance with the Right-to-Know Standard and can exact penalties and fines for failure to comply. Basically, inspections can occur for five reasons:

1. Employee complaints
2. Fatalities
3. Inspections of high-hazard facilities such as chemical, manufacturing, and construction companies
4. Catastrophes (five or more employees hospitalized)
5. General inspections (announced or unannounced)

Although it is true that OSHA most often inspects facilities that belong to high-hazard industries, the preceding reasons also may be used to justify inspection of smaller facilities.

In addition to compliance requirements, implementing a hazard communication program also provides a strong foundation for hazardous materials management. For example, the MSDSs and the hazardous chemical list required by the Hazard Communication Standard allow for easier tracking of chemicals when they become waste. Additionally, employees already will be trained in where to go for information and how to protect themselves.

☐ Laboratory Safety Standard

The Laboratory Safety Standard (29 CFR 1910.1450) was issued by OSHA on January 31, 1990, to address the hazardous substances found in all laboratories. This standard establishes the requirement for developing and implementing a chemical hygiene plan covering each laboratory using hazardous chemicals.

The Laboratory Safety Standard contains all the elements of the Hazard Communication Standard, as well as a number of elements specific to the laboratory environment. Because this is a specialized standard specific to laboratories, questions concerning this standard should be referred to the facility's laboratory department. The chemical hygiene plan should be included in the facility's safety policy manual.

☐ State Right-to-Know Laws

As OSHA was developing a Hazard Communication Standard, many states remained uncertain as to the final results. To deal with their chemical hazard concerns promptly, a number of states enacted their own right-to-know laws. This added to the complexity of compliance because some state laws were stricter than the federal standard and have remained so. On the other hand, many states adopted the federal standard in its entirety; therefore, compliance with the federal standard is sufficient for facilities in those states. It is important to know the regulations of the state in which a facility is located.

☐ Hazardous Chemical Waste Safety Program

After their use, hazardous chemicals become hazardous wastes. However, as such, they still pose risks to the facility and the environment. They must be contained appropriately and stored under the proper conditions. Most important, facilities cannot dispose of these wastes in a haphazard manner. Improper disposal can pollute the environment and endanger the life and health of people and wildlife, and can result in fines being levied against the facility.

The Environmental Protection Agency (EPA) has the power under several laws to prevent such damage to the environment. The law of primary interest to health care facilities is the Resource Conservation and Recovery Act (RCRA). Health care facilities must realize that they generate hazardous waste in quantities significant enough to be covered by RCRA. Xylene, azides, formaldehyde, and mercury represent just a few of the waste chemicals that health care facilities produce in everyday operation and whose disposal is covered by RCRA.

Definition of Hazardous Waste

According to RCRA, a discarded material is a hazardous waste if it meets certain criteria. These include:

- The material appears on one or more hazardous substance lists published by the EPA.
- It has any of the characteristics listed in figure 6-3.
- It is an acutely hazardous waste as defined by the EPA (for example, cyanide and cyanide compounds, arsenate and arsenic compounds, sodium azide, parathion, osmium tetroxide).

Determination of Generator Status

The health care facility must conduct a survey to determine the quantity and type of hazardous wastes it produces. From this, it determines its generator status. The EPA recognizes the following categories of generators:

- *Conditionally exempt generator:* Up to 100 kg of nonacutely hazardous wastes per month
- *Small-quantity generator:* Between 100 kg (220 lbs) and 1,000 kg (2,200 lbs) of non-acutely hazardous wastes per month
- *Large-quantity generator:* Greater than 1 kg (2.2 lbs) of acutely hazardous wastes per month and greater than 1,000 kg of nonacutely hazardous wastes per month

Each category has specific EPA regulations that health care facilities must understand. Most health care facilities fall into the small-quantity generator category, generating between 100 and 1,000 kg (2,200 lbs) of nonacutely hazardous waste per month. Each facility must determine its own category and understand the regulations that apply.

Figure 6-3. Hazardous Waste Characteristics

Characteristic	Definition	Examples
Ignitability	Easily combustible or flammable; with a closed cup flash point of less than 140 degrees Fahrenheit	Xylene, benzene, ethyl ether, acetone, methanol
Corrosivity	Dissolves metals, other materials, or has a pH of < 2 or > 12.5	Sodium hydroxide, hydrochloric acid, sulfuric acid
Reactivity (Explosive)	Unstable or undergoes rapid or violent chemical reaction with water or other materials, or has explosive characteristics	Examples: azides, hydrogen peroxide (30%), picric acid, perchloric acid (60%)
EP (Extraction Procedure) Toxic	May release toxic substances into groundwater or cause a poison hazard to human health or the environment	Compounds containing lead, mercury, chromium, silver, arsenic

Reprinted, with permission, from *Managing Health Care Hazards.* Chattanooga, TN: Chaff & Co., 1993, p. 2-2.

If a facility generates more than 100 kg of hazardous waste per month, it must obtain an EPA identification number. To obtain this number, the facility should contact the state hazardous waste management agency or the EPA regional office and ask for Form 8700-12. When the EPA receives the completed form, it will assign the facility a number.

Hazardous Waste Storage Requirements

RCRA strictly regulates storage containers and storage conditions. Its regulations include inspections, security, appropriate room condition maintenance, and accurate labeling.

Containers used to store hazardous waste should only be large enough to hold amounts for short periods. Once wastes have been contained, they may not be stored without a permit unless they are kept for fewer than 180 days for small-quantity generators that ship their wastes less than 200 miles for disposal, or 270 days for small-quantity generators that ship their wastes further than 200 miles.

Labeling

All waste containers must be clearly labeled. Labels must include the following:

- Proper DOT (Department of Transportation) shipping name describing the waste
- UN or NA number obtained from DOT files
- Generator information
- EPA ID number assigned to the facility
- EPA waste number from the DOT tables
- Accumulation start date
- Manifest document number

Standard DOT and EPA labels are available from many suppliers and label companies. Some disposal companies may require additional information. (See figure 6-4 for an example of a hazardous waste label.)

Hazardous Waste Reduction

Complying with the many specific requirements under RCRA may become complex, particularly for facilities with many different types and sources of waste. It is important to mention that an effective waste management strategy often overlooks waste reduction. However, every facility should have an ongoing program to reduce the amount of hazardous waste it generates.

One approach to waste reduction is through material recycling and reuse. For example, xylene, which is commonly used in histology labs, can be recovered by distillation, thereby reducing waste volume. However, due to vapors and explosion hazards, caution must be used in any recovery process such as distillation.

Another alternative is substitution. Increasingly, manufacturers are producing nonhazardous (or less hazardous) substitutes for products that previously contained hazardous chemicals. Department heads should contact the manufacturers or distributors of the chemicals or chemical compounds to determine if they have nonhazardous or less hazardous equivalents. The number of possible substitutions may be surprising, and even if they are more expensive, the cost probably will be made up in savings on waste storage, treatment, and disposal.

A frequently used way to reduce the amount of waste is neutralization or "de-naturing." This process converts hazardous substances to relatively harmless ones that can be disposed of in a routine manner, such as through the sewer system. The waste is neutralized by mixing it with another substance that renders it inert. For example, inorganic acids can be mixed with inorganic bases in the right amounts to nullify the acids. Although a number of resource books list such combinations and provide directions for mixing, only trained personnel and those familiar with the RCRA Standard should perform such mixtures. The local sewer district should be contacted to determine limits for disposal of neutralized substances.

Figure 6-4. Hazardous Waste Label

HAZARDOUS WASTE

FEDERAL LAW PROHIBITS IMPROPER DISPOSAL.

IF FOUND, CONTACT THE NEAREST POLICE, OR PUBLIC SAFETY AUTHORITY, OR THE U.S. ENVIRONMENTAL PROTECTION AGENCY.

GENERATOR INFORMATION:

NAME ____________________

ADDRESS ____________________ PHONE __________

CITY ____________________ STATE ______ ZIP __________

EPA ID NO. / MANIFEST DOCUMENT NO. ____________________ / __________

ACCUMULATION START DATE ____________________ EPA WASTE NO. __________

D.O.T. PROPER SHIPPING NAME AND UN OR NA NO. WITH PREFIX

HANDLE WITH CARE!

STYLE WM6

Printed by Labelmaster, An American Labelmark Co., Chicago, IL 60646 (800) 621-5808

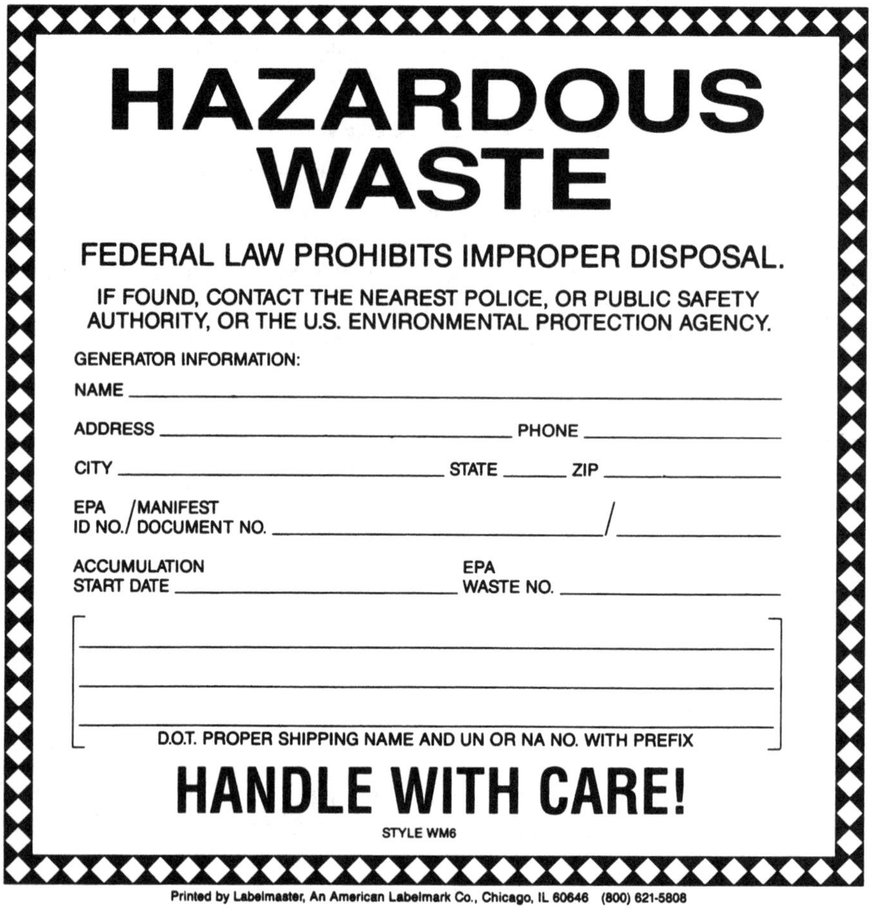

Source: Labelmaster Division, American Labelmark Co., Chicago.

Hazardous Waste Segregation

Too often, a nonhazardous material is not separated from hazardous waste before it is placed in drums to be discarded. The nonhazardous material is then labeled hazardous as well. This can greatly increase the amount of waste classified as hazardous and thus multiply the cost of treatment, transportation, and/or disposal. Therefore, it is important that hazardous waste be separated from other wastes. With good planning and waste reduction techniques, hazardous waste reduction can significantly reduce hazardous materials disposal costs.

Cleanup of Hazardous Material Spills

Spills of hazardous materials can occur anywhere in the health care facility. Although any hazardous material presents the opportunity for exposure, spills greatly increase that potential, often spreading or leaking into hard-to-reach areas. They can occur in rooms that are poorly ventilated, and their fumes can reach toxic or explosive levels of concentration. Small spills can be cleaned up by employees who regularly work with the material and are trained in the regulations of the Hazard Communication Standard. However, large spills—those requiring assistance from outside the work area—involve training beyond that required by the Hazard Communication Standard. Because of the dangers involved, OSHA has implemented a Hazardous Waste Operations and Emergency Response Regulation (CFR 1910.120) known as HAZWOPER. This regulation requires specific training in spill cleanup that will enable employees to do the job safely. Individuals involved in the spill response must be trained as required in the standard. Personal protective equipment (PPE) is almost always required, as is medical surveillance for the response team.

Examples of spills that may require assistance from individuals trained under the HAZWOPER Standard include:

- *Mercury:* Blood pressure units and thermometers can break and spill mercury that tends to break into small particles. In poorly ventilated areas, mercury vapors can reach toxic levels that require special cleanup techniques and PPE.
- *Ethylene oxide:* This hazardous material is used to sterilize medical and surgical supplies and equipment. Leaks during maintenance operations or in high-pressure supply lines are not uncommon and, depending on the amount spilled, can create hazardous conditions.
- *Formaldehyde:* Laboratories, pathology, and surgical units frequently use formaldehyde. It is a powerful reducing agent, and in the air it oxidizes to formic acid. Vapors are intensely irritating and high concentrations can be hazardous. Cleanup depends on the size of the spill, and requires knowledge of containment, neutralizing, and disposal methods.

Training spill response personnel is costly and time-consuming. Because large spills are not a common occurrence, the response team must practice very frequently so that it will know what to do and how to use the equipment when a large spill occurs. In the interest of saving time, money, materials, and personnel, the following is suggested:

- For spills of less than 500 cc that are not producing toxic fumes, department personnel should be trained in the use of appropriate spill kits and PPE that does not include the use of a self-contained breathing apparatus. All likely "spill areas" should be supplied with appropriate spill kits, disposal policies, and PPE.
- For spills greater than 500 cc, or any amount that produces toxic fumes, the area should be evacuated, other personnel kept out, the operator informed, and the public hazardous material response unit (usually a division of the fire department) called in. When this unit arrives, it should be provided with the MSDS for the chemical, a location map, and standby assistance. Most likely, the facility will still have to properly store and dispose of the hazardous waste created during the cleanup.

Cleaning up chemical spills can be dangerous and costly for the facility and the employees. Some facilities may opt to have only outside agencies clean up spills, others may choose to clean up everything, and still others may choose the method discussed above. Whatever the facility decides, policies must be written and reviewed, employees trained, and equipment available.

☐ Cytotoxic Drug Safety Program

Cytotoxic drugs, also called antineoplastic agents and chemotherapy drugs, are used in the chemotherapeutic treatment of cancer. They are designed to limit or reverse the growth of malignant tumors. To do this, many cytotoxic drugs must create change at the most basic level of cellular activity. The powerful potential of these drugs can make them very hazardous to individuals not being treated for cancer. In fact, in healthy individuals, cytotoxic agents have been linked to cancer, organ damage, sterility, and birth defects. In addition, acute effects include irritation of the skin and mucous membranes (especially the eyes), and tissue necrosis (the "death" of tissue).

Guidance and regulations for handling cytotoxic drugs come from several sources. Many cytotoxic drugs appear on EPA hazardous substances lists. OSHA has issued guidelines for the use of chemotherapeutic drugs. Moreover, OSHA's General Duty Clause (see chapter 2) requires employers to provide a safe and healthful workplace for employees. Harmful exposure to cytotoxic drugs could constitute a violation of this clause.

The health care personnel potentially exposed to chemotherapy drugs are many. They include physicians and employees from the following departments:

- Pharmacy
- Nursing
- Housekeeping
- Laundry
- Oncology
- Pathology
- Emergency department
- Morgue

Training in safe methods for handling cytotoxic drugs should be in place for all affected staff. In addition, detailed policies and procedures should be written for all tasks that pose the potential for cytotoxic exposure, including mixing the drugs, administering them, handling specimens from patients undergoing chemotherapy, disposing of chemotherapy drugs and contaminated waste, cleaning areas where patients receive chemotherapy, cleaning spills of cytotoxic drugs, and disposing of contaminated wastes. Although it is not possible within the scope of this book to discuss all the procedures for working with or around cytotoxic drugs, following are some helpful guidelines:

- The OSHA Instruction PUB 8-1.1, *Work Practice Guidelines for Personnel Dealing with Cytotoxic (Antineoplastic) Drugs* and the National Study Commission on Cytotoxic Exposure (NSCCE) guidelines for handling antineoplastic drugs should be consulted.
- All cytotoxic drugs and wastes should be labeled, and should be segregated from infectious and other chemical wastes. A yellow background with black lettering is becoming accepted as signifying cytotoxic waste. It helps distinguish cytotoxic drugs from "red-bagged" infectious waste.
- Syringes and needles should never be cut, and all sharps should be disposed of in a puncture-resistant container.
- The facility may wish not to allow pregnant or breast-feeding women to handle cytotoxic drugs at all.
- Urine and excrement from patients undergoing chemotherapy should be handled only when using proper PPE.
- Personnel handling cytotoxic drugs or wastes contaminated by cytotoxic drugs, including laundry and housekeeping personnel, should be required to wear appropriate gloves and approved protective disposable gowns.
- Employees should always wash their hands after handling cytotoxic drugs or cytotoxic-contaminated items, even if they wore gloves.
- Personnel mixing chemotherapy drugs should be provided with a Class II, Type A or B biological safety cabinet.
- Smoking, drinking, applying cosmetics, and eating in areas where these drugs are prepared, stored, or used should be strictly prohibited. Employees can ingest harmful amounts of the drug through any of these activities.
- Spills should be cleaned up immediately by a properly protected person trained in the appropriate procedures. Access to spill areas must be restricted.
- Most chemical inactivators can produce hazardous by-products and should not be applied to the spilled cytotoxic agent/drug.
- All contaminated surfaces should be thoroughly cleaned with a detergent solution and then wiped clean with water.

Cytotoxic drugs can have serious effects on exposed individuals, including long-term consequences that may not appear for years or even decades. To avoid the potentially tragic conditions associated with exposure and to reduce the facility's vulnerability to litigation, a thorough program of control and annual medical surveillance should be in place. This program will contribute significantly to the maintenance of a safe and healthful work environment. Policies should be kept in the safety manual, reviewed annually, and updated as necessary.

☐ Radioactive Materials Safety Program

Radioactive materials are used and stored in a number of locations throughout the facility. Departments where these materials are used most frequently include the following:

- Diagnostic radiology and radiation therapy (also called nuclear medicine or radiation oncology)
- Pathology laboratory
- Cardiology testing departments and cardiac catheterization units

Radioactive materials also are found in the facility in locations other than departments. These locations include:

- Waste radioactive material storage areas (used for storage of radioactive materials prior to disposal)
- Materials management and shipping (used for storage of incoming radioactive materials prior to delivery)

The Nuclear Regulatory Commission (NRC) and most state departments of health regulate the licensing, use, and storage of radioactive materials. The Department of Transportation regulates the shipping of radioactive materials and RCRA regulates the disposal of waste materials.

Accidents or incidents involving radiation are infrequent in health care facilities. Normally, the use of radioactive materials is confined to highly qualified technicians who have been trained to avoid overexposure.

☐ SARA Title III, or Community Right to Know

As previously discussed, through application of the Hazard Communication Standard and a thorough hazardous waste management program, harmful substances can be controlled as they enter, are handled within, and leave the facility. However, what happens when a hazardous substance is released into the environment, potentially spreading illness throughout the community surrounding the facility?

Chapter 2 introduced the Superfund Amendments and Reauthorization Act (SARA). Title III of SARA sets up a system whereby local communities engage in planning to prevent such accidents and to minimize their destructive effects should such an emergency occur. The act recognizes that only through cooperation between businesses and the community can there be an effective and coordinated response to emergencies involving hazardous chemicals.

The primary responsibility for health care facilities under Title III is in the area of emergency planning. Often referred to as Community Right to Know, Title III requires states to designate emergency planning districts, along with emergency planning committees for each district. These committees plan an organized response to be undertaken in the event of an environmental disaster. Committees include wide-ranging representation such as the media, community groups, health personnel, and fire protection representatives.

The planning committees begin by identifying businesses that use, store, transport, or generate certain large quantities of hazardous materials. To help plan what will be done to treat those affected by a release of hazardous substances, hospitals near these businesses must provide representation to the local emergency planning committee. They must assist in identifying routes for transporting the sick and injured, and protective measures for paramedics and other personnel. They also must develop a disaster preparedness plan for accommodating and treating large numbers of those made ill by the substance. Hospitals must be aware that they could be called to participate in this valuable community planning process. The health care facility also may be a user, generator, transporter, or storer of hazardous materials (for example, ethylene oxide). If so, the quantities, locations, and so on must be reported to the local SARA emergency planning commission.

☐ Conclusion

The use of hazardous materials in health care facilities presents a multitude of risks. A hazard communication program provides the basis for managing chemicals as they enter and are used in the facility, hazardous waste regulations manage the chemicals once they become waste, and Title III protects the community from the hazardous effects of the substances through a planned response to an environmental disaster. When properly implemented, these programs form an interlocking process that serves to protect the safety and health of employees, patients, and the surrounding community.

Bloodborne Pathogens

Every day, health care workers provide compassionate care for patients suffering from illnesses and emergencies. These workers protect and save lives, treat the sick, clean rooms, discard waste, and in the process of performing their duties may be exposed to the risk of contracting diseases from bloodborne pathogens. Although there are many different pathogens, hepatitis B virus (HBV) and human immunodeficiency virus (HIV) are the most likely of the serious viruses to affect health care workers. HBV weakens the liver, causing flulike symptoms, and can be fatal. HIV, which causes AIDS, attacks the immune system and leads to death.

In response to growing concern over the transmission of the HIV/HBV viruses, the federal Occupational Safety and Health Administration (OSHA) moved to enact the Occupational Exposure to Bloodborne Pathogens Standard (1910.1030). Commonly called the Bloodborne Pathogens Standard, it is intended to limit occupational exposure to blood and body fluids and other potentially infectious materials, because any exposure could result in the transmission of bloodborne pathogens and lead to disease or death. A number of states with state OSHA programs have adopted regulations more stringent than the federal OSHA standard, and health care facilities in these states should assess their compliance with the state standard.

This chapter describes the principal requirements of the Bloodborne Pathogens Standard and what health care facilities must do to ensure their compliance with the standard. A glossary of terms is included as an appendix at the end of the chapter.

☐ Requirements of the Bloodborne Pathogens Standard

The Bloodborne Pathogens Standard covers all employees working in the health care facility who could reasonably be expected to come in contact with blood and body fluids and other potentially infectious materials. A performance-oriented standard, it is designed to give employers flexibility in developing worker protection programs that are unique to particular settings and consistent with its intent. Compliance with the standard is the cornerstone for preventing exposure to infectious diseases, and hazard surveillance techniques used to evaluate facility compliance with traditional safety standards also can be used to evaluate compliance with the Bloodborne Pathogens Standard, specifically with regard to universal precautions and engineering controls.

To effectively carry out a compliance monitoring program, it is essential to understand the requirements of the Bloodborne Pathogens Standard. Following are six things facilities must do in order to comply with the standard's principal requirements:

1. Develop an exposure control plan
2. Minimize exposure risks to employees

3. Provide voluntary hepatitis B vaccination to employees at risk of exposure at no cost to employees
4. Communicate the hazards posed by bloodborne pathogens
5. Document and investigate all incidents to prevent future incidents
6. Maintain records for employee training, vaccination, vaccination declination statements, and postexposure medical evaluations

Develop an Exposure Control Plan

The Bloodborne Pathogens Standard requires employers to develop an exposure control plan in which tasks and procedures and job classifications where occupational exposure to blood and body fluids occurs, or could occur, are identified and listed in writing, without regard to personal protective clothing and equipment. Lists are designated "A" for high risk and "B" for low risk. The plan also must set forth the schedule for implementing other provisions of the standard, and specify procedures for evaluating compliance and investigating circumstances surrounding exposure incidents. Additionally, the plan must be made accessible to employees and available to OSHA; and employers must review and update it at least annually to accommodate workplace changes.

Minimize Exposure Risks

The standard mandates universal precautions (in other words, treating all blood and body fluids/materials as if infectious), emphasizing engineering and work practice controls. It also stresses hand washing, and requires employers to (1) provide hand-washing facilities and (2) ensure that employees use them following exposure to blood and body fluids. Further, the standard requires the employer to institute procedures to minimize needle sticks, minimize the splashing and spraying of blood and body fluids, ensure appropriate packaging of specimens and regulated wastes, and either decontaminate equipment or label it as contaminated before shipping it to servicing facilities.

Additionally, the standard requires employers to provide, at no cost to employees, appropriate fluid-resistant personal protective equipment (PPE) such as gloves, gowns, masks, mouthpieces, and resuscitation bags, which employers must require at-risk employees to use. Further, employers are responsible for cleaning, repairing, and replacing PPE as necessary. In addition to cleaning following contact with blood and body fluids or other potentially infectious materials, the standard requires the facility to use a written schedule for cleaning and for identifying the method of decontamination. It specifies methods for disposing of contaminated sharps, and sets forth standards for containers for these items and other regulated waste. The standard also includes provisions for handling contaminated laundry to minimize exposure.

The facility should adopt the philosophy that monitoring for compliance with this standard is the same as monitoring for compliance with any other regulation discussed in chapter 2. This philosophy especially applies to engineering and work practice controls, exposure incident investigation, PPE, and recordkeeping. For example, engineering and work practice controls include the following stipulations:

- Sharps containers must be available in all locations where employees handle or could come in contact with needles and other sharp items.
- Used needles and other sharps must be kept in puncture-resistant containers, and containers should not be overflowing.
- Warning labels must appear on containers of regulated waste.
- Containers of infectious waste must not show signs of leakage during storage, handling, and shipping.
- Work areas must be kept clean.
- Spills must be cleaned up.

- Universal precautions must be adhered to.
- Food must be segregated from potentially infectious materials.

Provide Hepatitis B Vaccinations

Hepatitis B vaccinations for all employees who may have occupational exposure to blood and body fluids must be made available within 10 working days of assignment. The vaccine must be available at no cost, at a reasonable time and place, under supervision of a licensed physician/health care professional, and must be administered according to the latest recommendations of the U.S. Public Health Service (USPHS). Prescreening may not be required as a condition of receiving the vaccine. At-risk employees must sign a declination form if they choose not to be vaccinated, but may later opt to receive the vaccine at no cost. Should booster doses later be recommended by the USPHS, employees must be offered them under the same conditions as the original HBV vaccine series.

Communicate the Hazards Posed by Bloodborne Pathogens

Warning labels, including the orange or orange-red biohazard symbol shown in figure 7-1, must be affixed to containers of regulated waste, refrigerators and freezers, and other containers that are used to store or transport blood or other potentially infectious materials. However, there are certain circumstances under which labeling can be forgone within the facility. These include:

- When blood or other potentially infectious materials are stored in containers such as red bags
- When universal precautions are used in the handling of all specimens
- When universal precautions are used in the handling of all laundry
- When blood that has been tested and found free of HIV or HBV is released for clinical use
- When regulated waste has been decontaminated

OSHA recognizes that under universal precautions, blood and body fluids and other potentially infectious materials from all source individuals are treated as if they contain HIV or HBV. However, the standard does not require that the infective status of source individuals or patients be identified. Additionally, OSHA believes that using labels to designate the bloodborne infection status of some individuals, and not others, sets up a dual system in which employees may take fewer precautions.

The communication of hazards posed by bloodborne pathogens includes requiring all employees with potential occupational exposure to participate in a training program during working hours. Training must be provided upon initial assignment and at least annually thereafter. Employees who have received appropriate training within the past year need only receive additional training in items not previously covered with specific reference to new exposures or procedures found in another facility. A complete bloodborne refresher program must occur

Figure 7-1. Biohazard Symbol

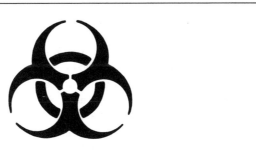

Source: Labelmaster Division, American Labelmark Co., Chicago.

annually. Additional training is required when changes or modifications of tasks or procedures occur, or when procedures affect the employee's occupational exposure.

Training programs must provide relevant information. Following are the principal elements to be included in training sessions:

- Where employees can obtain a copy of the standard and an explanation of its contents
- How diseases are transmitted
- The employer's exposure control plan and how employees can obtain a written copy of it
- Means of recognizing tasks that may involve exposures
- Methods of preventing exposures through engineering and work practice controls and the use of protective equipment
- Proper use and handling of PPE
- Facts on the hepatitis B vaccine
- Action to take in an emergency situation
- How to report exposure incidents
- Information on postexposure evaluation and follow-up
- Explanation of signs and labels
- The opportunity for questions and answers

Document and Investigate Incidents

The standard specifies procedures that must be made available to all employees who have had an exposure incident. In addition, any laboratory tests must be conducted by an accredited laboratory at no cost to the employee. The medical evaluation must be made available immediately after the exposure incident. The exposed employee should report to the appropriate health care professional within 72 hours if emergency treatment is not indicated. Follow-up must include:

- Confidential medical evaluation documenting the circumstances of exposure
- Identification and testing of the source individual, if feasible
- Testing of the exposed employee's blood, if he or she consents
- Postexposure prophylaxis
- Counseling
- Evaluation of reported illnesses

Health care professionals must be provided with specified information to facilitate their evaluation and written opinion on the need for hepatitis B vaccination or other medical procedures following exposure. Information such as the employee's ability to receive the hepatitis B vaccine must be supplied to the employer. All diagnoses must remain confidential. Figure 7-2 provides a flow diagram to determine if postexposure testing of the exposed employee is indicated.

Recordkeeping

The standard requires that medical records be kept for each employee with occupational exposure for the duration of his or her employment plus 30 years. The records must be kept confidential, and must include name, social security number, hepatitis B vaccination status (including dates), results of any examinations, medical testing and follow-up procedures, a copy of the health care professional's written opinion, and a copy of all information provided to the health care professional. Additionally, training records must be maintained for three years, and must include dates, contents (or a summary) of the training program, the trainer's name and qualifications, and names and job titles of all persons attending the sessions.

Medical records must be made available to the subject employee, anyone with written consent of the employee, OSHA, and the National Institute of Occupational Safety and Health (NIOSH). Medical records are *not* to be made available to the employer. Disposal of records must be in accordance with OSHA's standard covering access to records.

Like other puncture wounds, needle sticks are considered injuries for recordkeeping purposes. Only those work-related injuries that involve loss of consciousness, restriction of work or motion, or medical treatment are required to be recorded on the OSHA 200 form. For example, needle sticks, lacerations, or splashes requiring medical treatment (such as gamma globulin, hepatitis B immunoglobulin, hepatitis B vaccine) must be recorded. In addition, because this type of treatment is considered absolutely necessary and must be administered by a physician or licensed medical personnel, such an injury cannot be considered minor. If an exposure incident results in a diagnosis of seroconversion, it must be recorded on the OSHA 200 Log as an injury (for example, "needle stick" rather than "seroconversion").

☐ Conclusion

The enactment of the Bloodborne Pathogens Standard was a significant step toward reducing the risk to health care workers of contracting infectious diseases. The requirements of the standard are similar to those of the Hazard Communication Standard, which addresses exposure to hazardous chemicals. Both standards require awareness training, engineering controls, and

Figure 7-2. Employee Exposure Flowchart

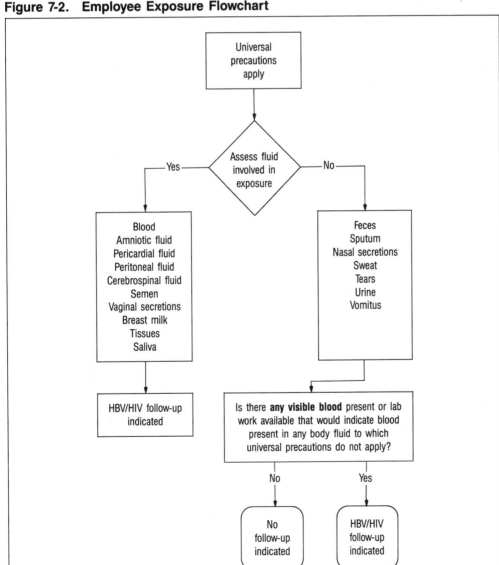

(Continued on next page)

Figure 7-2.   (Continued)

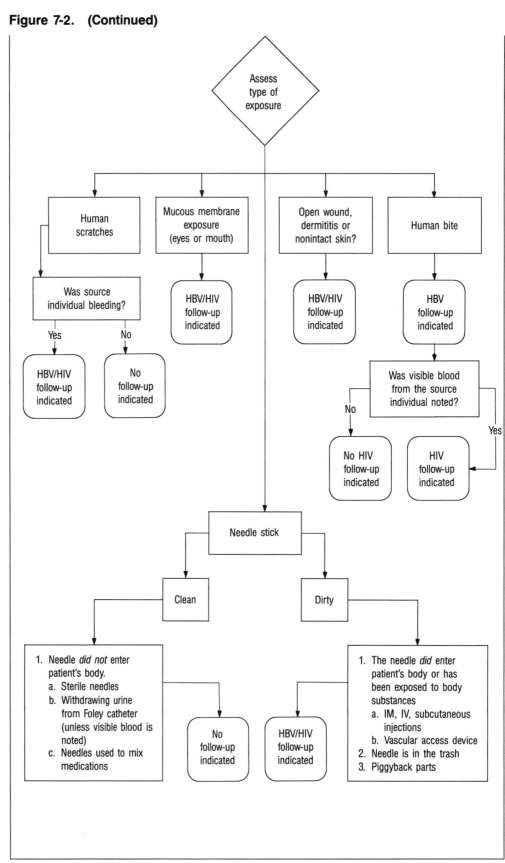

Reprinted, with permission, from *Managing Health Care Hazards.* Chattanooga, TN: Chaff & Co., 1993, pp. 3-4–3-5.

the use of PPE as ways to avoid exposure to hazardous materials. However, the Bloodborne Pathogens Standard has additional requirements, including providing HBV vaccination and postexposure testing and follow-up. Because of the serious consequences of contracting infectious diseases, health care facilities must not only implement the standard's requirements, but also ensure continuing compliance by the use of aggressive monitoring and evaluation procedures.

☐ Glossary

Blood: Human blood, human blood components, and products made from human blood.

Bloodborne pathogens: Pathogenic microorganisms present in human blood that can cause disease in humans. These pathogens include, but are not limited to, hepatitis B virus (HBV) and human immunodeficiency virus (HIV).

Contaminated: The presence, or the reasonably anticipated presence, of blood and body fluids or other potentially infectious materials on an item or surface.

Contaminated laundry: Laundry that has been soiled with blood and body fluids or other potentially infectious materials or that may contain sharps.

Contaminated sharps: Any contaminated objects that can penetrate the skin including, but not limited to, needles, scalpels, broken glass, broken capillary tubes, and exposed ends of dental wires.

Decontamination: Use of physical or chemical means to remove, inactivate, or destroy bloodborne pathogens on a surface or item to the point where they no longer are capable of transmitting infectious particles and the surface or item is rendered safe for handling, use, or disposal.

Engineering controls: Controls (for example, sharps disposal containers, self-sheathing needles) that isolate or remove the bloodborne pathogens hazard from the employee.

Exposure incident: A specific eye, mouth, other mucous membrane, nonintact skin, or parenteral contact with blood and body fluids or other potentially infectious materials that results from performance of an employee's duties.

Hand-washing facility: Facility providing an adequate supply of running potable water, soap, and single-use towels or hot-air drying machines.

HBV: Hepatitis B virus.

HIV: Human immunodeficiency virus.

Occupational exposure: Reasonably anticipated skin, eye, mucous membrane, or parenteral contact with blood and body fluids or other potentially infectious materials that may result from performance of an employee's duties.

Other potentially infectious materials:
- Human body fluids, including semen, vaginal secretions, cerebrospinal fluid, synovial fluid, pleural fluid, pericardial fluid, peritoneal fluid, amniotic fluid, saliva in dental procedures, any body fluid that is visibly contaminated with blood, and all body fluids in situations where it is difficult or impossible to differentiate between body fluids
- Unfixed tissue or organs (other than intact skin) from humans (living or dead)

- HIV-containing cell or tissue cultures, organ cultures and HIV- or HBV-containing culture medium or other solutions; and blood, organs, or other tissues from experimental animals infected with HIV or HBV

Parenteral access: Piercing mucous membranes or the skin barrier through events such as needle sticks, human bites, cuts, and abrasions.

Personal protective equipment (PPE): Specialized clothing or equipment worn by employees to protect against a hazard. General work clothes (uniforms, pants, shirts, blouses) not intended to function as protection against a hazard are not considered to be PPE.

Regulated waste: Liquid or semiliquid blood and body fluids or other potentially infectious materials; contaminated items that would release blood and body fluids or other potentially infectious materials in a liquid or semiliquid state, if compressed; items caked with dried blood or other potentially infectious materials and capable of releasing these materials during handling; contaminated sharps; and pathological and microbiological wastes containing blood and body fluids or other potentially infectious materials.

Research laboratory: Laboratory producing or using research-laboratory-scale amounts of HIV or HBV. Research laboratories may produce high concentrations of HIV or HBV but not in the volume found in production facilities.

Source individual: Any individual, living or dead, whose blood and body fluids or other potentially infectious materials may be a source of employee occupational exposure. Examples include, but are not limited to, hospital and clinic patients, clients in institutions for the developmentally disabled, trauma victims, clients of drug and alcohol treatment facilities, residents of hospices and nursing homes, human remains, and individuals who donate or sell blood or blood components.

Sterilization: Use of a physical or chemical procedure to destroy all microbial life including highly resistant bacterial endospores.

Universal precautions: An approach to infection control. According to the concept of universal precautions, all human blood and certain human body fluids are treated as if known to be infectious for HIV, HBV, and other bloodborne pathogens.

Work practice controls: Controls that reduce the likelihood of exposure by altering the manner in which a task is performed (such as prohibiting recapping of needles by a two-handed technique).

Waste Disposal

As the growing problem of waste disposal gains greater media and legislative attention, health care facilities continue to search for more cost-effective means of disposal. The ideal solution would be one that is acceptable to the public, meets regulatory requirements, reduces liability, and makes no unreasonable financial demands on the facility.

Once the health care facility has collected its hazardous chemical and regulated medical wastes, it must choose between on-site and off-site disposal for each waste type. Some facilities prefer incineration of certain medical waste streams, whereas others prefer to use off-site contract disposal firms. Some facilities prefer to ship hazardous chemical waste for disposal, rather than recover it through distillation or some form of treatment. However, regardless of the disposal method chosen, the facility must be aware of the many regulations that apply to all disposal options. In addition, cost and liability issues come into play in making the final choice.

This chapter covers disposal issues concerning both hazardous chemicals and regulated medical wastes. It also examines disposal regulations concerning radioactive waste.

□ Disposing of Hazardous Chemical Waste

Hazardous chemical waste (discussed in chapter 6) may be treated on-site, disposed of on-site, or disposed of off-site. The following subsections discuss these options.

Treating Hazardous Chemical Waste On-Site

Some forms of treatment can be used on-site to convert hazardous waste to a nonhazardous form. For example, inorganic acids can be mixed with inorganic bases to neutralize the acids. According to Environmental Protection Agency (EPA) regulations, hazardous chemical wastes may be treated in this manner without a special permit, provided the facility follows certain requirements. The facility must:

- Treat the accumulated hazardous waste within 180-270 days, depending on shipping distances
- Comply with container regulations
- Take steps to prepare for and prevent accidents

If the facility does not meet these requirements and wishes to treat hazardous waste on-site, a hazardous waste treatment permit must be obtained. However, some states have regulations that are more restrictive and prohibit treating on-site without a permit, even when the facility meets EPA requirements.

Disposing of Hazardous Chemical Waste On-Site

The facility may not dispose of waste on-site unless a disposal permit has been obtained. However, the EPA states that under certain circumstances certain types of waste may be legally disposed of without a permit. For example, certain wastes may be disposed of by discharging them directly into the sewer drain. However, this is not considered good management practice, and in many states or communities, this practice may be illegal. For information concerning wastes that may be disposed of in this manner, the local waste water treatment office or state hazardous waste management agency should be contacted.

Disposing of Hazardous Chemical Waste Off-Site

Although disposal of hazardous waste off-site would appear to offer an easy alternative to on-site disposal, it carries with it significant responsibility. This responsibility is primarily one of accurate recordkeeping and choosing licensed transporters and disposal sites.

Maintaining records of how the generated hazardous waste is handled is a critical part of avoiding problems with regulatory requirements. This is because one of the major reasons for passage of the Resource Conservation and Recovery Act (RCRA) was to establish a "cradle-to-grave" management system for hazardous waste. That is, Congress wanted the EPA and the states to be able to trace any shipment of hazardous waste created by the generator through the process of transportation and eventual handling by treatment and disposal facilities.

The cradle-to-grave concept involves use of the following:

- *Identification numbers:* Every site where regulated wastes are generated must be identified on the EPA's computer system by an EPA ID number. This number allows the EPA and the states to keep track of the kind of waste being generated and its source.
- *Hazardous waste manifest:* This manifest is a shipping form that identifies the following:
  —The type and amount of waste being transported off-site
  —Who is generating the waste
  —Who is transporting the waste
  —Where the waste is going

The manifest also satisfies the requirements of the Department of Transportation (DOT) for shipping papers to accompany hazardous waste shipments. Once the hazardous waste shipment has reached its destination, a signed copy of the manifest is returned to the facility. A system must be set up to ensure that the signed manifests are returned within 45 days, as specified by RCRA regulations. If necessary, follow-up action must be taken to ensure that the manifests are returned within the allotted time frame. One way to do this is to call the transporter about the manifests if they are not returned within 30 days.

Even after the hazardous waste is shipped off-site, the facility remains potentially liable for any mismanagement of the waste. The manifest tracks the waste during shipment and provides acknowledgment that no problems occurred along the way. It also provides an important means of demonstrating the facility's compliance with the law. Together, the identification number and the shipping manifest offer the means to set up a waste file that will provide a paper trail for use in proving compliance and avoiding future liability.

When EPA or state agencies conduct inspections, one of the first things they look at is the hazardous waste file. If there is no hazardous waste file, or if the records are disorganized, the inspector may become suspicious about how the facility is handling regulatory requirements. Therefore, it is essential to set up an orderly hazardous waste file in order to avoid experiencing RCRA noncompliance and cleanup liability.

☐ Disposing of Regulated Medical Waste

Regulated medical waste (discussed in chapter 7) also may be disposed of on-site or off-site. The following subsections examine these disposal options.

Disposing of Regulated Medical Waste On-Site

Disposing of medical waste safely, economically, and within government guidelines is becoming increasingly more complex. Some of the more frequently used methods, such as incineration and autoclaving, are drawing increased public scrutiny, as well as greater regulatory involvement. On the other hand, off-site disposal of treated waste into municipal landfills is being prohibited much more frequently by state and local governments. Therefore, facilities must make the difficult decision between treating medical waste on-site or shipping it to a hazardous waste management facility.

Many facilities are finding that on-site disposal, using newer technologies as well as some of the older approaches that have been improved upon, is offering sound alternatives to the off-site options. These alternatives include:

- Thermal (includes autoclaving, incineration, microwaving, electrothermal radiation, infrared heating, and lasers)
- Chemical (includes gaseous or liquid disinfectants and encapsulation systems)

Many factors must be considered in choosing alternate waste treatment technologies. Figure 8-1 lists issues that must be carefully weighed and prioritized, considering the needs of the individual facility and community.

Because of the number of issues to be evaluated, facilities often employ consultants to perform the analysis necessary to reach a decision on the type of waste treatment best suited to the facility. In addition to other factors, consultants compare on-site disposal with the cost of off-site disposal and provide expertise to make sure that all government air pollution regulations are met.

Disposing of Regulated Medical Waste Off-Site

Unlike the RCRA cradle-to-grave concept and the DOT manifest and tracking system, medical waste disposal is regulated by each state with widely varying requirements. In addition, the federal DOT does not require the manifest and tracking system for medical wastes. Rather, shipping requirements are regulated on a state-by-state basis.

Figure 8-1. Issues for Evaluating Alternate Waste-Treatment Technologies

Technical Issues

- Effectiveness of treatment
- Degree of residue destruction

Legal Issues

- Regulatory requirements
- Permitting processes

Community Relations Issues

- Public acceptance
- Owner/operator accountability

Equipment Issues

- Vendor qualifications/capabilities
- Installation requirements
- Size/space considerations
- Ease of use
- Reliability (guarantees and warranties)

Operational Issues

- Capacity
- Waste segregation/handling
- Waste classes that cannot be treated
- Worker safety concerns

Economic Issues

- Capital costs
- Operational costs (for example, energy)
- Maintenance costs
- Labor costs

Environmental Issues

- Air emissions
- Effluents
- Energy sources

Reprinted, with permission, from *Managing Health Care Hazards.* Chattanooga, TN: Chaff & Co., 1993.

Therefore, it is essential that each facility understand its state regulatory requirements. Most states require records of the amount of medical waste generated, and this and other requirements are detailed in the waste permit. It is important to read the permit carefully in order to avoid compliance problems.

The greatest concern for a facility is the possibility that regulated medical waste will be disposed of improperly, incurring fines or public relations problems. This concern is no different from that faced in the disposal of hazardous chemical waste. The best way to prevent these problems from occurring is to use the same principles of recordkeeping required by RCRA and DOT regulations. In addition, a qualified waste transporter and disposal firm must be chosen.

☐ Disposing of Radioactive Waste

Several enforcement agencies regulate disposal of radioactive wastes. The primary controlling agency is the Nuclear Regulatory Commission (NRC). Some radioactive waste may be kept on-site for extended periods, allowing the radioactivity to decay to safe levels and then be disposed of in a sanitary landfill. Some isotopes are provided by nuclear pharmacies that will pick up the waste after its use. Other radioactive wastes may need to be stored and transported to a regulated radioactive material disposal facility. Radioactive wastes sent to disposal sites must be tracked and documented to ensure proper disposal. Records must be kept permanently and are subject to audit by federal, state, and local agencies.

☐ Choosing Qualified Waste Transportation, Treatment, and Disposal Contractors

Many facilities contract with a firm, or firms, to transport, treat, store, and/or dispose of some of their waste. Because the generator potentially retains liability for its waste, even after the waste leaves the facility, great care should be exercised in selecting a reputable and experienced contractor.

The facility should begin looking for a contractor by contacting state environmental agencies for a list of disposal firms. Other sources include other health care facilities, industry groups, or associations that may be willing to recommend contractors they have used; trade journals and organizational magazines; and telephone directories.

Several steps should be followed in choosing a qualified contractor. The facility should:

- Conduct a brief telephone interview
- Evaluate the company's financial stability
- Consider the services the company offers
- Determine whether the company's insurance coverage is adequate
- Contact the company's references
- Obtain descriptions of previous jobs performed (The contractor should have some health care experience.)
- Check with environmental officials on the firm's background and compliance history
- Secure the right documentation
- Interview the candidate one-on-one
- Obtain a proposal, checking for the necessary elements
- Review the contract for the responsibilities it gives the contractor and any liabilities it may leave for the generator
- Monitor and stay involved in the contractor's work

□ Conclusion

Health care facilities are faced with the increasingly difficult task of choosing waste disposal options. They must choose between on-site and off-site disposal for each type of waste they generate, and must follow the requirements for proper disposal issued by federal, state, and local agencies. Additionally, they must consider a number of issues in choosing alternate waste disposal approaches, including technical, legal, community, and economic issues. And finally, because facilities remain liable for their waste until, and in some cases after, it is properly disposed, sound procedures for choosing qualified waste transportation, treatment, and disposal contractors are essential. Throughout the process, health care facilities must adopt a cradle-to-grave philosophy in managing disposal of their regulated waste.

Fire Safety

An organized system of fire safety is a vital component of the health care facility's safety program. Because fires are always a possibility, the facility must have an aggressive fire safety program based on comprehensive policies and procedures. To prevent fires from occurring, fire prevention practices such as good housekeeping and arson awareness should be stressed. Should a fire occur, detection and fire suppression systems should be in place to provide an immediate response.

Another important factor in the fire safety program is that of developing a productive working relationship with the local fire department. A fire department representative should be invited to attend safety committee meetings and can serve as a source of information on codes and fire prevention techniques. Additionally, this individual can help plan drills and in-service training.

This chapter describes the minimum fire safety guidelines for health care facilities set forth by regulatory agencies and state and local laws. It also discusses fire prevention methods and the importance of developing a master fire plan.

☐ Fire Safety Requirements

The National Fire Protection Association (NFPA) (see chapter 2), along with its two most important codes for health care—NFPA 99, Standard for Health Care Facilities, and NFPA 101, Life Safety Code, is considered the authoritative source on fire safety. In addition, requirements set forth by NFPA are complemented by Joint Commission on Accreditation of Healthcare Organizations (JCAHO) fire safety standards and Occupational Safety and Health Administration (OSHA) regulations pertaining to employee safety. These standards and regulations, together with local and state laws, provide the basic guidelines for fire prevention. Following are some of the most important requirements for health care facilities:

- Patient care buildings must comply with state and local codes and the appropriate edition of the Life Safety Code. A comprehensive statement of construction and fire protection must describe this compliance. However, the facility may adopt "equivalent" measures as long as they are as effective as, or more stringent than, the applicable code.
- The facility must have a written fire plan documenting measures used to prevent and respond to a fire. All fire protection measures must be documented in policies and procedures.
- Manual fire alarm stations and a fire detection system must be installed in each building. The detection system should automatically activate an alarm in the event of fire. Fire department notification also must be provided.

- Manual fire alarm stations must be located near each required exit and at other locations, so that travel distance does not exceed 200 feet.
- All fire alarm and detection systems must be tested at least quarterly.
- Heating and air-conditioning ducts and related equipment must be installed in accordance with NFPA requirements.
- The fire alarm must be distinct from other paging codes and loud enough to be heard over normal operational noise. Visual signals should be provided for the hearing impaired in accordance with the Americans with Disabilities Act (ADA).
- Electrical monitoring devices of automatic sprinkler systems must be connected to the fire alarm system. These must be tested at least annually.
- Fire extinguishers must be clearly identified and appropriate for the type of fire likely to occur in the areas in which they are located. (See figure 9-1 for descriptions of fire extinguisher classifications.) Fire extinguishers must be inspected at least monthly and maintained in accordance with NFPA 10.
- New items such as mattresses, drapes, furnishings, or floor coverings should be checked by the safety director to ensure that they meet the proper flame and smoke spread ratings. Many of these items may be treated with a fire-retardant material. Staff must be advised that dry cleaning can remove the fire-retarding finish and that the finish must be reapplied before the materials are returned for use.
- Wastebaskets must be made of noncombustible materials.
- Sections of privacy curtains within 18 inches of the ceiling in sprinkler-protected patient care areas must have a minimum of ½-inch mesh. Recent testing indicates that the sprinkler head dispersion pattern is severely hampered by curtains of fine mesh. All other areas protected by sprinklers must maintain a clearance of 18 inches from the bottom of the sprinkler head to the top of any materials being stored.
- Personnel must be trained and educated regularly in all facets of fire safety.
- Fire drills must be conducted quarterly for all personnel on all shifts, including personnel at outlying clinics.
- A facilitywide smoking policy should be developed and enforced.
- Electrical safety procedures must be written and enforced.

Figure 9-1. Fire Extinguisher Classifications

Types of fire extinguishers in health care facilities correspond to three categories of fires. Each class of fire extinguisher should be used only on the kind of fire for which it was designed. For example, using a Class A extinguisher, which is meant for ordinary combustibles, on an electrical (Class C) fire can be extremely dangerous. All extinguishers must therefore be clearly labeled according to their classifications, and staff should be trained in recognizing and using the different types.

Class A: Class A fires involve ordinary combustible materials such as wood, paper, cloth, rubber, and many plastics. Class A extinguishers rely on water-based solutions, Halon (when the extinguisher has 9.5 pounds or more of Halon in it), or multipurpose dry chemicals. These extinguishers should be identified by a green triangle containing the letter *A*.

Class B: Class B fires involve flammable and combustible liquids, greases, oils, tars, oil-based paints, lacquers, and the like. This type of fire also involves flammable gases. A fire involving a flammable gas should not be extinguished until the gas source has been shut off. With Class B fires, smothering the fire to interrupt the supply of air is most effective, so Class B extinguishers employ such substances as foam, Halon, multipurpose dry chemical, dry chemical, or carbon dioxide. These extinguishers are labeled with a red square containing the letter *B*.

Class C: Class C fires are located in or near live electrical equipment. Here an extinguishing agent that will not conduct electricity is needed. Thus, Class C extinguishers utilize carbon dioxide, Halon, or dry chemical. These extinguishers are marked with a blue circle containing the letter *C*.

Class ABC: This type of fire extinguisher is capable of fighting Class A, B, or C fires. It can be useful to prevent confusion. However, ABC extinguishers may leave a residue, so personnel may want to use a CO_2 or Halon extinguisher around equipment that may be damaged by the powder-type extinguishers. Multipurpose extinguishers are marked with the letters *A, B,* and *C*.

- The emergency power system must provide electricity to the following systems in the event of an outage:
  —Blood, bone, and tissue storage units
  —Emergency care areas
  —Emergency communication systems
  —Exit illumination
  —Fire alarms
  —Fire detection systems
  —Fire pumps
  —Medical air compressors
  —Medical/surgical vacuum systems
  —Nurseries
  —Obstetrical delivery rooms
  —One elevator
  —Operating rooms
  —Postoperative recovery rooms
  —Special care units
- Elevators traveling 25 feet or more above the level where fire-fighting personnel will enter must be equipped with an automatic elevator recall system. (Section 7-4 of NFPA's Life Safety Code further explains this requirement.)
- Commercial cooking equipment must be installed with proper systems to remove grease-laden vapors in accordance with NFPA 96. Gas and electric cooking equipment protected by an automatic extinguishing system should be equipped with an automatic shutoff device to stop the flow of gas or electric current.
- Linen and rubbish chutes must be kept in good repair. Doors must shut and lock when released. In addition, chutes must be protected by an automatic fire suppression system such as automatic fire sprinklers. Chute construction should be in accordance with NFPA 82, *Incinerators, Waste and Linen Handling Systems and Equipment*.
- The fire protection program must be reviewed and revised regularly. Solutions to problems must be determined, implemented, and documented.

These represent minimum fire safety requirements. State and local governments often promulgate their own codes, which may be stricter than OSHA regulations or JCAHO and NFPA rules. Facilities should check with state and local authorities and the local fire department to determine what additional standards will affect them. (See figure 9-2 for a fire safety inspection checklist.)

☐ Fire Prevention Methods

Prevention methods include good housekeeping, proper storage of hazardous materials, smoking restrictions, arson awareness, and so on. Procedures should be developed and employees trained in fire prevention to reduce the frequency of fires.

Housekeeping

Housekeeping is one of the foremost lines of defense against fire. Carelessly discarded rags that have been in contact with flammable liquids such as gasoline or cleaning fluids have been known to cause fires in health care facilities. In addition, improperly stored hazardous materials, piles of linens in corridors, obstructed sprinklers or fire doors, cluttered work areas, and accumulated trash all can start fires or encourage their spread.

To help avoid fires, every employee should be held accountable for keeping work areas clean and orderly. Additionally, housekeeping personnel should be directed to respond promptly to spills and not allow rubbish to accumulate. A clean and orderly facility will prevent many fires and inhibit the spread of any that start.

Figure 9-2. Fire Safety Inspection Checklist*

Sprinkler and Fire Detection System

_____ Sprinkler system serviced annually by qualified agency.

_____ Sprinkler valves accessible (with no recently stored material forming obstructions) and sealed open.

_____ Sprinkler valves operate easily. No leaks, corrosion, or other defects noted in system.

_____ Sprinkler water flow alarm tested.

_____ Fire detection (alarm) system tested.

Fire Alarm Facilities

_____ Location signs in place.

_____ Boxes unobstructed.

_____ Date of last test: _____

_____ Auxiliary boxes have sign indicating whether system is connected to fire department.

Fire Doors

_____ Operative.

_____ Unobstructed (no wedges to hold doors open).

Fire Hose (Standpipes)

_____ Cabinet door operative.

_____ Hose condition satisfactory (not rotted, wet, moldy, and so forth).

_____ Nozzle in place; proper type.

_____ Hose properly hung in rack; aired; rehung to avoid creases.

Fire Extinguishers

_____ All extinguishers mounted in properly designated locations.

_____ Extinguisher seals intact and inspection tags properly initiated. To be inspected monthly, and serviced at least once a year.

_____ Proper decals or other markings on extinguisher and wall to indicate type of fire on which extinguisher can be used.

_____ No leaks, corrosion, or other defects noted.

_____ Extinguishers unobstructed, ready for instant use.

_____ No carbon tetrachloride or other vaporizing liquid used in any extinguisher.

_____ Personnel informed on proper use.

Exits and Exitways

_____ All exits clearly marked and exit lights on.

_____ All exit lights clean and of proper wattage.

_____ Exitways free from obstructions.

_____ Furniture placed so that occupants can quickly and safely evacuate rooms.

_____ Exterior grounds kept clear of objects that might impede evacuation of fire-fighting equipment.

Stairways

_____ Doors at each level operate satisfactorily and are kept closed.

_____ Stairways free of obstructions.

_____ Landings properly lighted.

Fire Drills

_____ Date of last fire drill: _____

_____ All employees and staff members participate in drill.

Auxiliary Lighting

_____ Auxiliary emergency generator operative: maintenance and operating condition.

_____ Fire door properly maintained.

_____ Lighting checked weekly; date of last test: _____

Figure 9-2. (Continued)

Smoking Regulations

_____ All smoking regulations met and enforced.

Electrical Wiring and Equipment

_____ All electrical equipment purchased and installed is tested for performance and safety.

_____ Appliances properly grounded.

_____ All motors of proper size; clean, free of lint; cords not frayed; grounded.

_____ Only qualified electricians are allowed to install or extend wiring.

_____ Use of extension cords discouraged. When their use is absolutely necessary, they should be checked to ensure they are not frayed or covered with grease or lint; length not over 10 feet; no multiple or "octopus" wiring connections to wall outlets; no cords under rugs or fabrics.

_____ All electrical circuits properly fused: 15 amp for general lighting circuits; 20 amp or more for special circuits.

_____ Emergency lighting system operable.

_____ Electric motors, fans, heaters, appliances, and fluorescent and other light fixtures free of combustibles; all such equipment easily accessible for replacement.

Heating, Ventilation, Flues, and Vents

_____ Air-conditioning equipment filters clean.

_____ Heating plant checked and serviced by qualified agency (annually).

_____ Flues and vents free of dust and obstructions. (See *Kitchen.*)

_____ Fire door operating in boiler room and incinerator room.

_____ No combustible storage in room.

Housekeeping, Storage, and Waste Disposal

_____ Brooms, mops, rags, and other cleaning supplies stored properly in metal cabinets or approved cans.

_____ Paints, solvents, thinners, and other flammables stored in metal cabinet; oily rags in metal safety containers.

_____ Combustibles kept clear of stove, heating appliances, heating plant, and water heater.

_____ Dry leaves, shrubbery trimmings, and other combustibles kept away from buildings.

_____ No combustibles stored under stairways.

Kitchen

_____ Hoods, vents, fans, and ducts in good condition and free from grease.

_____ Hood filters cleaned regularly; date of last cleaning: _____

_____ Hoods equipped with appropriate automatic extinguishing devices.

Surgery and Obstetrics

_____ Monthly record readings of conductivity of surgery floor and furnishings, to check degree of insulation resistance.

_____ Proper relative humidity (R.H.) maintained.

_____ Mechanical ventilation adequate.

_____ Equipment grounded, properly maintained, and tested periodically.

_____ Rules and regulations posted.

Alcohol, Ether, and Similar Chemicals

_____ Properly stored.

_____ Properly dispensed.

_____ Flammables should be stored in refrigerators designed and approved for this purpose.

_____ No Smoking signs provided.

(Continued on next page)

Figure 9-2. (Continued)

Compressed Gases (Nonflammable)

_____ Cylinders properly capped and stored in designated area.

_____ Cylinders properly secured by chain or strap to wall.

_____ Storeroom vented to outside.

_____ Fire door operative.

_____ No Smoking signs provided.

Miscellaneous Hazards

_____ Nonsmoking areas equipped with adequate signs.

_____ All curtains, draperies, and decorative fabrics in exitways treated with flame retardant.

_____ Everyone in every department has been warned never to use flammable fluids for cleaning floors, clothes, or furnishings.

_____ Gasoline is kept for use with power mower or generator; is properly located in safety can with self-closing cap.

_____ Target areas such as mechanical equipment rooms, storage and supply rooms, and the laundry receive surveillance beyond routine checks for malfunctions and fire hazards.

*This inspection checklist is a guide. Items should be added or deleted in accordance with the size and operation of the particular facility. Each feature is to be checked monthly unless a different interval is indicated.

Smoking Regulations

The JCAHO prohibits the use of smoking materials throughout hospital buildings unless there is a written physician's authorization. This policy provides a more healthful environment and reduces the risk of fire.

Arson Awareness

Arson is a serious problem, and many officials believe it is difficult to detect and relatively impossible to prevent. However, certainly one way to help prevent arson is to increase employee awareness of it. Arson can be committed by anyone, regardless of age or sex. Disgruntled patients or employees, and psychiatric patients pose a risk of arson because they seek attention or revenge.

Arsonists will set fires anywhere they believe they are alone and unobserved. Fires may be started in wastebaskets, broom closets, mattresses, and so on. Therefore, it is important that places with low activity levels be either locked or regularly monitored in order to discourage arson.

Employees are the best arson deterrent in the health care facility. They should examine work areas for conditions that may be attractive to an arsonist. For example, roll-away beds left in corridors or stacks of empty boxes are convenient materials for an arsonist to use. All flammable liquids and housekeeping supplies must be secured. Employees should be alert to anyone hanging around secluded areas and immediately report any suspicious behavior to security.

☐ Master Fire Plan

In addition to fire prevention, the facility must have procedures for responding to fires in a safe and orderly manner. Health care facilities must have a way to protect patients while guarding employee safety and minimizing property damage. These procedures, and the fire safety program in general, must be outlined in the facility fire plan. The JCAHO requires that the plan address the fire safety needs of the entire facility. Factors that should be included when developing the master fire plan include the following:

- Fire response training
- Fire drills
- Command decisions
- Fire brigade or fire response team
- Evacuation

Fire Response Training

Along with fire prevention methods, employees should be taught emergency response procedures. The proper response, immediately carried out, can go a long way toward reducing damage and injury. Many health care facilities use acronyms to ensure that even under the strained emotional conditions evoked by fire, employees will remember the steps to take. For example, one acronym used by health care facilities is RACE. It stands for four steps that employees should follow during a fire. These are:

1. **R:** *Remove* everyone from immediate danger.
2. **A:** Turn in the *Alarm* followed by a phone call. Turning in the alarm is a definite priority because the fire department can be on its way while other activities are being performed. Thus, while one employee is turning in the alarm, another can be removing a patient, employee, or visitor from danger.
3. **C:** *Confine* the fire. All doors and windows should be closed to prevent the spread of smoke and flames.
4. **E:** *Extinguish* the fire. This should only be done in the case of a manageable fire, such as a fire in a wastebasket. Immediately available equipment such as a blanket, sheet, or bedside water pitcher should be utilized to extinguish the fire. If possible, two employees should fight the fire together using two fire extinguishers.

Some facilities print the acronym on the back of employee name badges or post it in prominent locations throughout the facility.

Fire Drills

Fire drills are a major component of fire safety training. They offer the opportunity to familiarize employees with proper fire plan procedures. For example, employees can:

- Implement the steps of the emergency response procedure
- Use the facility's emergency number to call the operator
- Extinguish a small fire by bringing a fire extinguisher to the scene of the fire

The JCAHO requires that fire drills be conducted at least quarterly and include all personnel on all shifts, including those working at outlying clinics. It recognizes real fires as drills as long as responses are documented and problems are addressed. These drills may include facilitywide fire drills and those limited to particular departments. Drills can be preplanned, giving staff members the opportunity to think about what their responses should be, or unexpected, giving the opportunity to assess reactions to a situation similar to a real fire. Regardless of the type of drill, it is essential that all employees be involved, including second-shift, third-shift, and outlying clinical staff.

Fire drills are used to test employee knowledge and provide information to correct employee deficiencies through retraining. During a fire drill, employees should be able to:

- *Recognize a fire drill and respond rapidly.* Some facilities use a blinking lantern, a marked flag, an announcement over the public address (PA) system, or personal notification of one or more employees to begin a drill.

- *Implement the steps of the emergency response plan.* While implementing these steps, employees can:
  - —Use dummies to practice removing someone from danger (nearby patients should be told what is occurring)
  - —Telephone the switchboard, identify themselves, give the location of the fire, and explain that it is a drill (unless the drill was preplanned and publicized)
  - —Wait for the fire response team, fire brigade, or fire department to arrive if information was given that the drill would involve a large fire
  - —Demonstrate knowledge of fire extinguisher location and use
- *Realize the facility fire page will be transmitted on the PA system along with the fire's location.* This means that the administrator or designee has been alerted to the fire and that the fire response team or fire brigade has responded to the alarm by heading toward the fire.
- *Wait for more information or the order to evacuate.* Employees should follow master fire plan procedures for ambulatory, semiambulatory, and bedridden patients when evacuating. They should work rapidly but not rush and, after evacuation, wait for the all clear signal or orders to evacuate further.

All fire drills must be documented. Fire drill documentation and evaluation is used to measure employee performance at the scene of the fire and facilitywide. Usually, security officers or safety committee members are responsible for documenting the response to the drill. If an educational program was conducted at the scene of the fire, employees should sign a document stating they were there for the training. Forms or checklists can be used to summarize response times, confusion noted, and areas for improvement. Documentation elements could include the following:

- Did the employee who encountered the fire follow the steps of the emergency response plan?
- Did designated personnel carry out their responsibilities correctly?
- Did employees in the area of the fire bring a fire extinguisher to the scene?
- Did employees in the area telephone the operator using the emergency number?
- What was the response time of the fire response team or fire brigade?
- Was evacuation rapid and orderly?
- Did alarm systems work correctly?
- Did all fire protection equipment used function correctly?

Employees should be questioned on how they viewed the drill and ways for improvement. In the accreditation process, the JCAHO will randomly sample employees, asking them to describe their role in the fire plan. Employees also may be asked to locate fire protection equipment and any equipment used to transport patients to safety.

Finally, fire department personnel should be involved in the whole process. They may direct the drill and should participate in its evaluation. Methods to improve performance may be suggested and should be implemented by the facility. Well-planned and regularly evaluated fire drills provide the key to a rapid, orderly response during a real emergency.

Command Decisions

During a fire, command decisions must be made that include the need for evacuation, internal and external communication, and liaison with the fire department. To accomplish this, members of the administration and other designated members should perform a number of procedures. They should:

- Gather in a preestablished command center.
- Announce the fire code slowly and clearly over the PA system, stating its location.

- Notify the fire department of the type and location of the fire. This is a secondary notification, because the first notification is the result of pulling a fire alarm or activating any part of the fire detection system.
- Dispatch a designated person to meet the fire department at a designated entrance and to secure an elevator designated for their use.
- Request that all telephone calls and nonemergency pages be held.
- Assess the progress and magnitude of the fire and keep all departments apprised.
- Notify the fire chief or senior fire officer of the need to evacuate the building.
- Announce the all clear after receiving it from the fire chief or the senior fire official.

Figure 9-3 lists examples of departmental responsibilities during a fire.

Fire Brigade

Some facilities establish a fire brigade to provide fire response. The brigade can rescue anyone in danger, sound the alarm if it has not yet been pulled, and fight the fire. Further, it can act as an excellent fire protection resource. Administration appoints the fire brigade team leader who in turn interviews and appoints brigade members.

Fire brigade members require training equivalent to that of fire fighters, such as using hoses and a self-contained breathing apparatus, rescuing trapped individuals, and administering first aid. A fire brigade must be trained to meet the OSHA Standards on Fire Protection (29 CFR 1910.156). Training must be well documented and every member must meet the same training requirements regardless of position on the team. If a brigade is established, OSHA requires employers to provide a written policy establishing the existence of the fire brigade.

The fire brigade's duties should be developed for each facility based on site-specific requirements and needs. These duties may include evacuation, fire suppression, fire control, and salvage operations, and should be developed in coordination with the local fire department.

The fire brigade may respond to two types of fires. These are:

1. *Incipient-stage (beginning) fires:* These are small fires that are limited to a well-defined area and do not yet threaten the structure of the facility.
2. *Interior-structural fires:* These are large fires that threaten the structure of the facility.

Employers must provide fire brigade members with appropriate personal protective clothing and equipment, at no cost to the employees, and must adequately maintain this equipment.

Fire Response Team

The fire response team is a group of employees trained to fight incipient-stage fires. Immediate action by the fire response team can limit or even extinguish an incipient-stage fire before the fire department arrives.

The fire response team is not a fire brigade and is not trained to meet the OSHA Standards on Fire Protection. Therefore, the fire response team must not fight interior structural fires.

Evacuation

Because complete evacuation to the outside is rarely necessary, it usually is not the first step of an evacuation plan. Total hospital evacuation is very involved and requires development of a regional plan that incorporates aspects of sheltering agreements with other facilities to accept patients and the availability of area emergency medical service (EMS) vehicles to accomplish evacuation. The need to continue vital patient care should be balanced against the degree of immediate fire threat. The facility administrator or designee will issue the order to evacuate in coordination with the fire department.

Figure 9-3. Fire Plan Responsibilities for Individual Departments

Nursing Units

Before a fire occurs:

1. One person should be designated to turn on all corridor lights.
2. One person should be assigned to monitor the telephone to answer emergency calls or relay messages.
3. One person should be responsible for ensuring that all room doors are closed.
4. A list of patients should be convenient to see that all are accounted for.
5. Every nurse should become familiar with the facility fire plan.

In the event of a fire:

1. Carry out immediate emergency response.
2. Clear exits and elevator area. Do not allow elevators to be used.
3. If fire is in your area, ensure that all oxygen in operation is shut off in a safe manner. Oxygen shut-off valves are located _____ . The (title) will make the decision as to when oxygen operation will be shut off.
4. If fire is not in the area, nursing managers should be prepared to use their personnel to care for patients transferred to the area or dispatch personnel to other areas.
5. Reassure patients who may become disturbed by the commotion.

Department Managers

Before a fire occurs:

1. Become familiar with the facility fire plan.
2. See that employees in their departments have been instructed as to their respective duties in case of fire.

In the event of a fire:

1. See that these duties are carried out.
2. Immediately upon hearing the alarm, ensure that all doors and windows in the area are closed.

Plant Services/Maintenance

Before a fire occurs:

1. Become familiar with the facility fire plan.
2. Ensure that designated members of the fire brigade or fire response team are thoroughly trained.
3. Assign one person on the 7 a.m.–3 p.m. shift to meet the fire department at a designated entrance and secure a designated elevator at ground level for their use.

In the event of a fire:

1. Carry out immediate emergency response.
2. The director of maintenance will report to emergency control center, as a member of the emergency control system.
3. Regulate air-handling equipment.
4. Secure electrical room, boiler room, and other maintenance areas, as necessary.

Housekeeping

Before a fire occurs:

1. Become familiar with the facility fire plan.
2. The director of housekeeping may assign, or be asked to assign, members to the fire brigade.

In the event of a fire:

1. Carry out immediate emergency response.
2. All other housekeeping personnel remain in their work areas and assist when directed.
3. If necessary, help remove any patient to a safe area.
4. On the 3 p.m.–11 p.m. shift, one person will be assigned to meet the fire department at a designated area and secure a designated elevator for their use.

Figure 9-3. (Continued)

Dietary

Before a fire occurs:

1. Become familiar with the facility fire plan.

In the event of a fire:

1. Carry out immediate emergency response.
2. If fire or smoke is in the area, turn off gas and electrical machinery.
3. Personnel are to remain in the department.
4. If necessary, remove any person to a safe area.
5. Await instruction from emergency control center and be prepared to assist wherever needed.

Laundry

Before a fire occurs:

1. Become familiar with the facility fire plan.

In the event of fire:

1. Carry out immediate emergency response.
2. If fire or smoke is in the area, turn off machines.
3. Personnel are to remain in the department.
4. Await instructions from emergency control center (described in detail in chapter 10) and be prepared to assist wherever needed.

All Other Departments

Before a fire occurs:

1. Become familiar with the facility fire plan.

In the event of a fire:

1. Carry out immediate emergency response.
2. Personnel are to remain in their departments.
3. If necessary, remove any person to a safe area.
4. Await instructions from emergency control center and be prepared to assist wherever needed.

Evacuation may be partial or complete and may be accomplished in two ways. These are:

1. *Horizontally:* This type of evacuation involves moving patients to a safe area on the same floor.
2. *Vertically:* This type of evacuation involves moving patients downward to other floors or to the outside using the stairs. Patients should be evacuated to higher floors only in emergency conditions.

Ambulatory patients should be assembled, instructed to form a chain, and then moved in a group. Semiambulatory patients should be assisted one-on-one as they are pushed in wheelchairs or walk. Finally, bedridden patients may have to be carried. (See figure 9-4 for descriptions of emergency patient carries.) Medical records should accompany patients. If this is not practical, records should be taken to a central location for distribution at a later date. Once safety has been reached, all patients need to be accounted for against the patient card file. The evacuation plan should end by detailing procedures for recovery—for example, how patients will be returned and what will be done with damaged areas.

☐ Conclusion

Health care facilities must develop a fire protection plan based principally on National Fire Protection Association guidelines. The plan must specify the fire prevention procedures that the

Figure 9-4. Patient Removal Methods

Infant and Child Removal

1. Place a blanket or sheet on the floor.
2. Place two infants in each bassinet, using diapers or small blankets for padding.
3. Place the bassinet in the middle of the blanket.
4. Use the baby vest if available or fold the blanket over one end, fold the corners in, then roll the sides in to form a pocket.
5. Grasp the folded corners of the blanket and pull the infants to safety. Two persons (or, if necessary, one person) can drag eight babies to the prescribed area.
6. Alternatively, place as many children as possible in one crib and pull the crib to the prescribed area.

Universal Carry

The universal carry is a method of removing a patient from a bed to the floor. It is a quick and effective method for removing a patient who is in immediate danger. This carry can be used by anyone regardless of patient size.

1. Spread a blanket, sheet, or bedspread on the floor alongside the bed, placing one-third of it under the bed and leaving about 8 inches to extend beyond the patient's head.
2. Grasp the patient's ankles and move the patient's legs until they fall at the knee over the edge of the bed.
3. Grasp each shoulder, slowly pulling the patient to a sitting position.
4. From the back, encircle the patient with your arms, place your arms under the patient's armpits, and lock your hands over the patient's chest.
5. Slide the patient slowly to the edge of the bed and lower him or her to the blanket. If the bed is high, instruct the patient to slide down one of your legs.
6. Taking care to protect the patient's head, gently lower the head and upper torso to the blanket and wrap the blanket around the patient.
7. At the patient's head, grip the blanket with both hands, one above each shoulder, holding the patient's head firmly in the 8 inches of blanket. Do not let the patient's head snap back.
8. Lift the patient to a half-sitting position and pull the blanketed patient to safety.

Swing Carry

The swing carry requires two trained persons.

1. One carrier, feet together, slides an arm under the patient's neck and grasps the patient's far shoulder. The carrier's free hand is slipped under the patient's other upper arm, grasping it, and taking one step toward the foot of the bed, the carrier brings the patient to a sitting position.
2. The second carrier now grasps the patient's ankles, bringing the patient's legs at the knee over the edge of the bed.
3. Each carrier takes one of the patient's wrists and pulls it down over the carrier's shoulder, supporting the patient's body.
4. Each carrier reaches across the patient's back, placing one carrier's free hand on the other's shoulder.
5. Each carrier reaches under the patient's knees to lock hands with the other.
6. Standing close to the patient, the carriers bring their shoulders up and remove the patient from the bed, carrying the patient to a safe area.
7. At the safe area, each carrier drops on the knee closest to the patient, leans against the patient, and rests the patient's buttocks on the floor. The patient's torso is lowered to the floor, and the patient's head is placed on a pillow or like protection. The patient's head must always be carefully protected.

Blanket Drag

If vertical or downward evacuation by an interior stairway is necessary, in many cases one person can handle a helpless patient by using the blanket drag.

1. Double a blanket lengthwise, place it on the floor parallel and next to the bed, leaving 8 inches to extend above the patient's head.
2. Using cradle drop, kneel drop, or other suitable means, remove the patient from the bed to the folded blanket on the floor alongside the bed.
3. Grasping the blanket above the patient's head with both hands, drag the patient headfirst to the stairway.
4. Position yourself one, two, or three steps lower than the patient, depending on your height and the patient's height. The patient's lower body inclines upward.
5. Place your arms under the patient's arms and clasp your hands over the patient's chest.
6. Back slowly down the stairs, constantly maintaining close contact with the patient, keeping one leg against the patient's back.

facility will implement as well as describe the facility's response in the event of fire. Because effective fire response depends on how well employees are trained, frequent fire drills are required to measure training effectiveness. The plan also must define the role of fire response teams or brigades, as well as how command decisions are made during a fire. Further, it must specify how patient and employee evacuation will be accomplished if required. Through employee training based on a well-defined fire plan and ongoing liaison with the local fire department, the risk of serious injury or damage to the facility will be greatly reduced.

Emergency Preparedness

I n the wake of a disaster, the community looks to its health care facility for assistance and information. Although the facility itself may have sustained significant damage, creating an immediate need to evacuate patients and nonemergency staff and volunteers, it must respond to the event by continuing to serve the community with as little impairment as possible. This can only be achieved through comprehensive, coordinated planning prior to an emergency. Staff members and volunteers must know their assigned roles and perform them rapidly and efficiently, and the facility must work in tandem with community agencies and volunteers. A carefully prepared and successfully implemented emergency plan is key to saving lives.

The facility must be prepared for excessive or unusual demands on its resources. An earthquake, hurricane, or tornado may not only result in an influx of critically injured people but also may prompt some victims to seek shelter and food at the facility. At the same time, the facility may still be reeling from its own disaster-related emergencies, such as building damage, fire, and power outage. For example, a severe winter ice storm may cause a total power outage in the community. A system must be in place that includes everything from keeping patients warm to preventing water pipes from freezing to adding sand to driveways for emergency vehicles. A comprehensive emergency plan prepares the facility to handle multiple emergencies by allocating resources to meet patient needs, continue service, and protect employees.

This chapter discusses the health care facility's need to identify potential disasters in its region and how to write an umbrella plan to facilitate its response to them. It also describes the importance of working with community resources to carry out its plan effectively.

☐ Identifying and Planning for Emergencies

Identifying and planning for emergencies requires the input of thoroughly trained individuals with emergency preparedness responsibilities. The process begins when the chief executive officer (CEO), in cooperation with the safety director, appoints an emergency preparedness coordinator and a committee (or staff may be invited to volunteer to serve on the committee). The committee can be small and often is a subsection of the safety committee. Representatives from departments that are vital in an emergency should serve as members. They should include medical staff, nursing administrators, physicians knowledgeable in emergency medicine, and personnel from security, safety, and engineering. The coordinator should be an individual knowledgeable in emergency planning and motivated to serve the facility in this capacity. With one person directly responsible for emergency preparedness, and a committee to support and assist that person, emergency planning gains direction and momentum.

As with other committees, individuals serving on an emergency preparedness committee need recognition for their participation. Recognition could be in the form of a certificate of appreciation, a plaque, or time off from other duties.

The facility's administration must allot sufficient time for the coordinator and the committee to create an emergency plan. Moreover, a solid plan may require items that are not presently in the facility's budget—for example, cellular telephones or walkie-talkies. Once the committee has determined what is needed to efficiently cope with a disaster, the items should be budgeted for and purchased as quickly as possible. Administrative support of the committee's decisions is a means of reinforcing the facility's commitment to the program.

In many parts of the country, certain types of disasters are unlikely to occur. Thus, the committee needs to concentrate on what is likely to occur at its particular location. For example, a facility in Kansas does not need to prepare for a volcanic eruption but should prepare for a tornado, whereas a facility near Mount St. Helens in Washington State would need to prepare for a volcanic eruption but not for a hurricane.

Types of Disasters

Because many types of disasters are possible, preparing for them is critically important. Earthquakes, tornadoes, hurricanes, and other natural disasters all require special emergency planning. A list should be made of all possible disasters within the facility's area, both natural and man-made, and a plan of action must be designed for each identified disaster.

The facility's planning efforts should include key personnel from local agencies. Following are some of the agencies that should be involved:

- Fire department
- Police department
- Power company
- Gas company
- Water company
- Telephone company
- Radio/television stations
- Local industrial safety specialists
- Local emergency planning committee
- American Red Cross
- Office of Emergency Services

Other emergencies may have risks that are not as widespread as those previously mentioned—for example, a chemical spill at a local industrial plant, a traffic accident involving a hazardous waste spill from a truck or train, a multiple-car accident, a train collision or derailment, a plane crash, a bomb threat, or a power outage. In addition, as the use of radioactive agents increases in various industries, an accident involving the release of a radioactive substance at a business or during a train or traffic accident is increasingly probable. Therefore, facilities near nuclear power plants are no longer the only ones who need a response plan for a nuclear incident. Some familiar occurrences, such as sudden and severe snowstorms, severe cold, or thunderstorms, also can spark an emergency situation in both the facility and the community.

An extremely important factor to consider is a backup emergency plan in the event that the facility itself is severely damaged or staff members are injured. There must be a plan and a method for immediately summoning off-duty staff members. An emergency such as an on-site water main break or a power outage would highly restrict the staff's ability to provide help to the injured. However, with a plan of action in place, the effects of structural damages or loss of services to the facility can be minimized so that the facility can continue to serve the community efficiently.

As a result, the emergency preparedness coordinator and the committee must approach emergency planning with an open mind. They must consider all the possibilities and build flexibility into the plan so that service can continue with minimal interruption. Further, they must recognize the increasingly wide variety of possible emergencies, as unfamiliar as they may seem. (See figure 10-1 for a list of possible emergencies that could affect health care delivery.) The

Figure 10-1. Potential Emergencies That Could Affect Health Care Delivery

- Train accident
- Epidemic of food poisoning or other illness
- Nuclear accident
- Internal fire
- Fire in the community
- Chemical spill or release
- Airplane crash
- Multiple-car collision
- School bus wreck
- Bomb threat
- Terrorist attack
- Hostage situation
- Strikes, picketing, protests
- Power outage
- Utility (water, heat, natural gas) failure
- Computer failure
- Earthquake
- Hurricane
- Tornado
- Blizzard
- Thunderstorm
- Drought
- Natural gas leak
- Building collapse
- Industrial or construction accident
- VIP disaster (for example, assassination or illness of a public figure)
- Flood
- Civil disturbance

Joint Commission on Accreditation of Healthcare Organizations (JCAHO) mandates the minimum number and types of disasters the facility must address through written policies and drills. At the least, these include fire, severe weather, civil disturbance, evacuation, bomb threats, loss of power or water, and hazardous material incidents.

Facility Risk Assessment

In identifying and planning for emergencies, the coordinator and the committee must consider several factors. For example, as mentioned previously, location of the facility has some bearing on the types of probable emergencies. As a result, the committee must conduct a risk assessment for its particular facility and locale. Is the facility near the ocean where hurricanes or tidal waves can develop? Is it in a part of the country that is predisposed to tornadoes, snow, drought, or frequent thunderstorms? Every geographical location and terrain bring their own unique possibilities for disaster or emergency.

Proximity to other institutions and businesses also can influence the type of emergency. For example, if the facility's grounds or roof include a heliport, planning for a plane crash will become a priority. If the facility is near a train station, train tracks, or a major highway, it must be prepared to deal with emergencies related to those types of transportation.

Equally important to consider are the types of businesses conducted in the community. Large manufacturing firms bring the increased possibility of a chemical release, a large-scale industrial accident, or a fire. In such cases, the facility must be prepared with toxicological data and special treatment methods.

Resource Planning

Another major factor to investigate is the resources of the facility. These include space, supplies, equipment, and staff. The facility must know beforehand what its capabilities are, rather than scrambling to take an accounting after disaster strikes. It is vital that the emergency preparedness coordinator and the committee take stock of the facility's resources in the course of designing the safety program.

Many questions should be asked by the coordinator and committee members to focus on the facility's needs. Key questions might include the following:

- What equipment is available, and what will be done if it is damaged?
- How long will it be until necessary supplies run out, and how will they be replaced?
- What staff services will be essential, and how will staff be called in?
- How many beds could be made available, and how quickly?

- What kinds of victims and how many could the facility accommodate? (For example, if the facility does not contain a burn unit, the plan should recognize that during a hotel fire in the area, many of the victims may have to be sent elsewhere for treatment.)
- What security or safety measures would be required?
- During an emergency, what are the risks to the facility, staff, and patients?

Different facilities have different resources and services, and making a list of them is a good way to begin formulating a successful emergency preparedness plan.

Routine maintenance of resources also is extremely important. For example, emergency power generators must be regularly started, tested, and serviced to ensure that electricity remains available. It should not be assumed that the backup generator will automatically work at peak efficiency during interruption of power. This assumption has often proven incorrect, and facilities have remained with limited or no electricity for weeks (sometimes months), greatly reducing the services the community so desperately needs in an emergency. Regular checks and maintenance can prevent such a frustrating and hazardous situation.

Another area of preparedness is planning how the facility will respond if it suffers partial destruction. Following are a few of the questions that will need to be addressed:

- How will food and water be given to patients?
- Should patients be evacuated to another facility? If so, how and to which facilities?
- Will the American Red Cross help with shelter?
- What about sufficient supplies of medication and the control of sanitation?

The committee must discuss how it can integrate with other community resources to maintain the highest quality of medical care possible during an emergency.

☐ Community Emergency Planning

Because disasters affect all sectors of the community, there often is a body within local government that oversees emergency planning. Frequently called the Office of Emergency Services (OES), this agency usually reports to the mayor or the county manager. It is responsible for planning and coordinating the response of community resources to an emergency.

One problem faced by community emergency planners is the lack of standard nomenclature for concisely describing the degree of an emergency. This lack of description can lead to serious problems for emergency management personnel. Often initial reports from the scene are greatly exaggerated and radio reports can be interpreted as "It's a big one, send everything you've got." A statement of this type could trigger a maximum response and even the recall of off-duty personnel. Even the news media can become involved in overstating the extent of the emergency. For example, surrounding emergency agencies hearing of the incident via the news media or police scanners may pitch in and send reinforcements. Within a short time, the disaster scene could be characterized not by a shortage of resources but by an overabundance of them. This poses additional strain on the already difficult problem of trying to organize and coordinate a large-scale response. Disaster researchers have described this type of scenario as "an informal mass assault."

Health care facilities also can be affected by the lack of communication regarding the extent of the emergency. At a confused disaster scene, many of those involved in the early care of disaster casualties believe the best action is to transport people to the nearest hospital. They may use any means at hand, such as police cars, taxis, buses, or by foot instead of in properly equipped ambulances. Often the nearest hospital is inundated with casualties. Those with lesser injuries typically arrive early at the hospital and in large numbers. Those who are more difficult to rescue, and who often have more serious injuries, arrive later at an already chaotic emergency department (ED). Concerned relatives flood hospital phone lines and make orderly communication with other treatment facilities impossible.

Several organizations are working to develop a simple, easy-to-use system to identify the scope of an emergency. One example is the system called PICE (Potential Injury Creating Event). PICE establishes a numerical code to be used in broadcasting an emergency. Each code represents a particular emergency and emergency description. The code also defines the exact status of an emergency, who should respond to the emergency, how they should respond, and so forth. (See figure 10-2 for a description of the PICE model nomenclature.)

☐ Utilizing Community Resources

Emergency preparedness is a cooperative venture between facility and community. Without this coordination, the disaster effort will be fragmented and ineffective. The community helps the facility through fire fighting, law enforcement, and ambulance services. On its side, the facility may respond to a communitywide disaster by providing on-site triage (a systematized procedure to assess casualty types, stabilize for transport, and coordinate transportation to appropriate health care facilities). In disasters that impair both facility and community (for example, a serious earthquake), the facility and the community rely on each other through a reciprocal relationship that benefits all involved.

During a disaster, there usually will be a demand on the facility from outpatients and other individuals who need access to their regular medical care or medication. A plan to divert these individuals to other medical resources in the vicinity (nursing homes, doctors' offices, medical clinics, and so on) will enable the facility to focus on the needs of emergency patients.

Figure 10-2. Example of the PICE System

To describe a disaster, choose a modifier from each of columns A, B and C in the table below:

Potential Injury Creating Event (PICE) Nomenclature

A	B	C	PICE Stage
Static	Controlled	Local	0
Evolving	Disruptive	Regional	I
Dynamic	Paralytic	National	II
		International	III

The meaning of the modifiers is as follows:

Column A describes whether there are ongoing problems.

Column B describes whether resources are overwhelmed and, if so, whether they must simply be augmented (disruptive) or must first be reconstituted (paralytic).

Column C describes the extent of geographic involvement.

Stage refers strictly to the chance that outside *medical* assistance will be required for the direct casualties of the disaster. For example:

- Stage 0 means there is no chance.
- Stage I means there is a small chance and outside help should be placed on "alert" status.
- Stage II means there is a moderate chance and outside help should be placed on "standby" status.
- Stage III means local medical resources are clearly overwhelmed and outside resources should be dispatched.

An example of the use of PICE nomenclature:

A multiple vehicle crash in a large city would be described as a static, controlled, local, PICE Stage 0.

Reprinted, with permission, from *Prehospital Systems and Medical Oversight*, A. E. Kuehl, Mosby Co., St. Louis, 1994, and modified with permission from K. Koenig and N. Dinerman.

This kind of coordinated effort does not occur unless a strong working partnership has been established prior to the emergency. Initiating and building a relationship represents a major goal for emergency planning. A cooperative relationship with the local fire department (see chapter 9) is crucial because fire can and often does occur simultaneously with other disasters.

SARA Title III, or the Community Right-to-Know Act (see chapters 2 and 6), is highly relevant to a facility's emergency preparedness. Under Title III, facilities near businesses that use large amounts of extremely hazardous chemicals must join a local emergency planning committee. Or if the facility itself uses large quantities of hazardous materials, it may be required to serve on the committee as a generator of such substances. Whatever the case, facilities involved in this planning should view their participation as an opportunity as well as a responsibility. Fire fighters, police, community officials, and the media also serve on the committee. By working closely with these individuals, facilities can begin to establish a cooperative relationship that will be essential to a coordinated and efficient response to all types of emergencies.

To foster communitywide cooperation, health care facilities should share emergency planning information such as emergency communication systems, evacuation procedures, and sheltering agreements. They also should cooperate with other health care facilities in community disaster drills and help evaluate each other's performance.

An important aspect of the interaction between health care facilities is mutual aid agreements. *Mutual aid agreements* are formal, written assurances that facilities will provide each other with well-defined services in specific emergency situations. For example, if a disaster exceeds the bed capacity of one facility, a second facility will take in the overflow. Or in the event of a citywide emergency, the written agreement could stipulate beforehand how many patients should be sent to each facility in the area.

Mutual aid agreements also should be used to set forth the relationship between the facility and other groups, such as the emergency medical service, the police, and the OES. The terms under which support may be offered or received should be spelled out clearly, along with the type of assistance to be provided, the estimated time that support will be necessary, and the way the agreement will be implemented. Each party should sign the agreement and include it as an appendix to its emergency preparedness plan.

Finally, there are many other sources of disaster planning information and assistance. Following are a few of them:

- Utility companies, to minimize the effect of an interruption in water, gas, telephone, or electrical service
- Local emergency medical services for initial treatment, triage, and transport of injured persons
- The National Disaster Medical System, which coordinates a national emergency preparedness program
- The Federal Emergency Management Agency (FEMA), for emergency assistance and information
- The National Weather Service, for severe weather warnings
- The National Oceanic and Atmospheric Administration, for information and support in planning for natural disasters

☐ Writing an Umbrella Plan

Once basic identification and planning have been accomplished, the emergency preparedness coordinator and the committee turn their attention to writing the plan. There should be a master (or umbrella) plan that lays out the foundation of the emergency response. However, although written plans are important, they are insufficient to ensure adequate preparedness. In fact, they can be an illusion of preparedness if they do not meet certain basic requirements. Written plans must be:

- Accompanied by adequate training
- Considered practical by the intended users
- Tied to the necessary resources
- Based on valid assumptions

Written plans that do not conform to these requirements tend to sit on the shelf and gather dust and are largely ignored in actual disasters because they do not fulfill real-world emergency response needs. This is one reason for the frequent observation that emergency response has occurred more in an ad hoc fashion than according to a plan.

The first step in preparing the plan is to gather information. This is done by asking questions and examining existing resources, including taking an actual tour of the premises. Notes should be taken, and a needs assessment list should be developed.

Once sufficient information has been gathered, the committee can begin writing the umbrella plan, incorporating certain crucial components. These include:

- A system of command
- A control center
- Methods of communication
- A system for mobilizing personnel/equipment
- An organized process of patient management
- A public information system
- Disaster drills

The following subsections describe these components.

System of Command

System of command refers to an organized hierarchy of control that is enacted immediately in an emergency. This system determines who can declare an emergency, convene the control center personnel, and order evacuation. A command system must include not only who is in charge of what but also who is second or third in command. Usually, the line of succession begins with the administrator in charge. If this individual is not available, responsibility transfers to the emergency preparedness coordinator, then to the chief of the medical staff, and so on. The chain of command, along with all other program elements, should take into consideration staffing shortages after normal working hours, on weekends and holidays, and at night. It also should acknowledge that those assigned certain emergency responsibilities may have been injured during the disaster or may be away from the facility at the time of the disaster. Having a system of command that is applicable in all situations prevents the chaos sometimes associated with the early stages of a disaster and activates the organized emergency response. The chain of command should list positions rather than names of individuals because the people filling those positions are subject to change.

Health care facilities must develop a command system that meets the needs of their organizational structure. However, there are command systems in place around the country that can be used for guidance. Most fire and police departments and the military have plans that may be useful. One system, the Hospital Emergency Incident Command System, has been developed specifically for health care facilities. It was developed through a joint effort of the Orange County Emergency Medical Services Agency and the State of California Emergency Medical Services Authority. A copy of the plan can be obtained from the Orange County agency listed in appendix A (at the end of the book).

Control Center

The control center is the designated place within the facility where decisions will be made. When an emergency situation arises, the administrator in charge declares an emergency, goes to the center, and summons the emergency control group. This group usually consists of an ED physician, the preparedness coordinator, the medical director, the director of nursing, the safety director, the director of engineering, and a public information manager. If these individuals are not available, designated department representatives should take their place.

The emergency control group forms a team that monitors the progress of the emergency, authorizes emergency actions, coordinates activities with other community agencies, and activates mutual aid agreements. In essence, along with the administrator in charge, team members control and coordinate the facility's emergency response.

The room the control group uses as its control center should be identified in the plan, but it may need to be changed depending on the damage to the facility. Yet another consideration when setting up a control center is whether the equipment is relatively portable. For example, following an earthquake that has caused structural damage to the facility, can the equipment be moved to another, safer part of the facility or to the parking lot in case of possible fire?

The control room should be close to the center of activity but far enough away from imminent hazards to maintain safety. It should contain copies of the plan, pencils and pens, an ample supply of paper, a typewriter, at least one direct-line telephone (in other words, one that does not go through a switchboard) and cellular phones or alternate communication systems (in the event lines are dead), telephone directories, tables and chairs, a transistor radio, a fax machine, and a supply of assorted sizes of batteries, blankets, and flashlights. The room chosen should be one that normally contains many of these items (for example, an office).

Communication

Communication between different areas of the facility and between the facility and the community is essential to a coordinated response. Switchboard personnel should be directed to keep all lines free except for emergency use, so that information can get in and out. To maintain outside communication, the facility should have a designated telephone line that does not go through the switchboard. In many disasters, however, outside telephone lines are not operational. Thus, the disaster plan must establish an alternate communication system. Short-wave (or ham) radio may be used for communication, and walkie-talkies can provide for interdepartmental conversation. The use of "runners" is another effective method of internal communication. Within the community, local ham radio clubs also can provide emergency communication during a disaster.

Mobilizing Personnel and Equipment

Employees whose services are crucial to successful emergency response must be listed, and a system for mobilizing them should be outlined in the plan. Following are some of the personnel to be included:

- Emergency department personnel, especially triage experts
- Engineering or maintenance personnel
- Nursing services personnel
- Medical staff, particularly specialists in injuries that may be prevalent (burns, asphyxia, crush injuries, radiation sickness, and so on)
- Security personnel
- Safety or risk management personnel
- Dietary personnel (to ensure provision of food)
- Switchboard personnel (if the telephone system is still operational)
- Housekeeping personnel (to move equipment and so on)

The plan should contain these individuals' names, home telephone numbers, and pager numbers. A priority calling list with alternate numbers also should be developed. People not involved in the immediate response (for example, support services staff) should be used as callers. The plan also should prepare the facility to transport these personnel if weather conditions make travel in personal vehicles difficult. Additionally, it should outline security procedures if rioting is involved. Identification cards should be provided in advance to key individuals to facilitate getting through police or security lines.

Patient Management

An organized process of patient management includes procedures and paths of evacuation, criteria for relocating patients to other facilities if the building has been severely damaged, a method for attending to visitors, and a system of triage by which incoming patients are prioritized according to the extent of their injuries. The patient management element also controls when, how, and which patients may be released to their families, if necessary.

Recordkeeping is important during a disaster. If there is a toxic spill that affects dozens—perhaps even hundreds—of people, they will need emergency attention. Under ordinary circumstances, when patients are admitted, there is always time for individual medical information to be completed on a chart. During an emergency, however, there is little or no time to take down the patient's medical history. The committee must anticipate that this may occur and have a means of swiftly obtaining the most critical information. This might be through the use of portable tape recorders, medical stenographers, or some other means.

These records also may influence federal government assistance to the affected area and indicate the impact so that future responses can be handled more efficiently. Data regarding how the emergency affected both the public and the facility can be extremely beneficial for several reasons. For example, without a data-gathering system in place, there would be no way to notify relatives of a patient's condition. In addition, transferring patients to another facility would be complicated.

Public Information

Public information is an important part of emergency response and one that often is overlooked. The media may be the facility's best (if not only) avenue for communicating critical information to the public. In many disasters, the facility experiences a barrage of media attention. To ensure that all information being released is accurate, information must come from a single source within the facility. For this reason, the emergency control group should include a public information manager. All staff members should be instructed not to answer questions from the press but, rather, to politely refer the press to the public information manager.

To prevent media personnel from interfering with the internal emergency response and to coordinate all information dissemination, an area should be designated to be the public information center. This area should be near the control center but, for obvious reasons, not be the same room. Like the control center, the public information center should be comfortable and stocked with chairs, pencils and pens, paper, a fax machine, a direct-line telephone, and perhaps a copier, snacks, and coffee. The public information manager should always remember that the way media personnel are treated often influences their coverage. Polite, respectful interactions with the media can enhance public perception of the facility's emergency efforts. The emergency preparedness coordinator should invite newscasters to tour the facility and introduce them to the public information officer. This public relations gesture would be appreciated and would let reporters know beforehand who their contact person will be in an emergency.

Disaster Drills

In some facilities, training for emergency preparedness is a requirement for nonmedical staff promotions and appointments to the facility's medical staff. Disaster drills represent one of the most effective ways to familiarize employees with the plan and allow them to practice their responsibilities. The JCAHO requires facilities to carry out drills and to document and evaluate them. Scenarios should be as realistic as possible. All employees should be encouraged to contribute to the evaluation, as should participating community agencies. The JCAHO may question employees randomly about the drill, including how it was evaluated. The entire emergency preparedness program should be reviewed by the safety committee each year and updated as facility capabilities or community needs change. All training, drills, and evaluations must be documented.

☐ Planning Specifically for Some Common Emergencies

In modern society, a number of social conditions and technological advances have become so widespread that they offer the potential of producing common emergency conditions. For example, computer systems are so widely used in industry that their breakdown produces an emergency situation that must be anticipated and prepared for. The following subsections provide tips for tailoring the health care facility's response to some specific emergencies.

Bomb Threats

Although bomb threats are not as common as some emergencies, unfortunately their increase in recent years in virtually all public institutions, including health care facilities, warrants development of an emergency plan. One important step in dealing with a bomb threat is to have the person receiving the call listen carefully and get as much information as possible from and about the caller. Figure 10-3 provides an example of a form to be filled out by the person receiving the call. This form, or a similar one, should be conveniently located at switchboards and other phone locations.

Once the information has been gathered and the telephone call has ended, the person who received the call should notify his or her supervisor. The supervisor in turn should inform the administrator, who then will notify security and the local police. As necessary, the administrator will activate the emergency control group. Depending on police protocol, searching should be initiated only with the help of the police. Searchers should be advised not to touch or move suspicious objects. The search should be called off as the time of detonation nears. With the help of the emergency control group, the administrator will give the order to evacuate. (The local police department should be contacted for more detailed instructions on dealing with bomb threats.)

Power Loss

The New York City blackout of 1977 illustrates the potential disaster caused by loss of electrical power. Although an outage in a health care facility cannot be compared to this citywide emergency, the provision of health care depends on electrically powered equipment, and a facilitywide power loss can take on disastrous proportions.

Again, it must be emphasized that regular inspections, testing, and maintenance of the emergency power generators should be a priority. However, disasters may damage these as well. Thus, it is important that the disaster plan include arrangements for renting or buying new generators. The facility should have a clear understanding with the company that supplies the generator(s) so that the company can respond quickly to the facility's needs. The plan also must outline ways for the facility to continue operating with limited power.

Strikes

Although not usually disastrous, strikes can cause disruption in services and may lead to violence. Unlike other emergencies, there is time to plan for a strike, because negotiations normally precede it. The administrator and emergency preparedness personnel should make use of this time to plan how vital services will be continued, how nonstriking personnel can be

Figure 10-3. Sample Response to Bomb Threat Form

RESPONSE TO BOMB THREAT

If you receive a bomb threat, you may be able to reduce the hazards in a real situation.

Instructions:

1. BE CALM; BE COURTEOUS; LISTEN.
2. DO NOT INTERRUPT THE CALLER.

Date _____ Time _____ Person receiving call_____.

Exact WORDS of person placing the call:_____
_____

Questions to Ask:

1. When is the bomb going to explode?_____
2. Where is the bomb right now?_____
3. What kind of bomb is it?_____
4. What does it look like?_____
5. Why did you place the bomb?_____

Try to determine the following:

Caller's Identity: ☐ Male ☐ Female ☐ Adult ☐ Juvenile Age____

Caller's Voice: ☐ Loud ☐ Soft ☐ High ☐ Deep ☐ Raspy
☐ Pleasant

Caller's Accent: ☐ Local ☐ Not Local Foreign Region_____

Caller's Speech: ☐ Fast ☐ Slow ☐ Distinct ☐ Disordered
☐ Stutter ☐ Slurred ☐ Lisp

Caller's Language: ☐ Excellent ☐ Good ☐ Fair ☐ Poor
☐ Foul ☐ Other

Caller's Manner: ☐ Calm ☐ Angry ☐ Rational ☐ Irrational
☐ Coherent ☐ Incoherent ☐ Deliberate
☐ Emotional ☐ Righteous ☐ Laughing
☐ Intoxicated ☐ Drugged

Background Noises: ☐ Office Machines ☐ Factory Machines
☐ Bedlam ☐ Train ☐ Music ☐ Quiet
☐ Voices ☐ Mixed ☐ Airplanes ☐ Party
☐ Street Traffic

Time Caller Hung Up:_____

Additional Information: _____

Action to take immediately after the call:

1. NOTIFY YOUR SUPERVISOR AND THE ADMINISTRATOR.
2. TALK TO NO ONE ABOUT THE CALL OTHER THAN INSTRUCTED BY YOUR SUPERVISOR.
3. BE PREPARED TO REPEAT SAME NOTIFICATION TO POLICE DEPARTMENT, AS REQUESTED.

Reprinted, with permission, from National Safety Council. *Long Term Care Safety Management Manual: A Handbook for Practical Application.* Chicago: National Safety Council, 1987, p. 114.

reassigned, where temporary replacement personnel for support services can be found, and other ways to deal with the strike.

Computer Failure

Health care facilities have displayed a rapidly growing reliance on computers for many tasks (other than record storage), such as admitting, ED information gathering, patient monitoring, and security systems. Although computers contribute greatly to the efficiency of operations, an institution's dependence on them leaves it vulnerable to computer failure and even sabotage—both of which are potentially disastrous in a health care setting.

All computer equipment should have a power-surge protective device. The facility should maintain an ongoing contract for the services of a repair firm (or firms) that agrees to respond immediately to any computer problems. The company also should be able to provide substitute equipment during lengthy repairs. The contractor, or a qualified staff member, should inspect the system and conduct preventive maintenance on a regular basis. Equally important, computer storage drives should be "backed up" periodically, and the backup floppy diskettes, tape, or optical disks should be stored off-site. Whatever site is chosen, it should be as fireproof as possible. Off-site storage reduces the possibility of losing months or years of data.

☐ Conclusion

Emergency preparedness is a major responsibility for all health care facilities and their personnel because they represent the guardians of health for the community and because the public looks to them for assistance and information in time of disaster. To provide the necessary assistance and information effectively, potential types of emergencies must be identified in advance and an effective umbrella plan, which can then be tailored to the individual emergency, must be written.

It should be understood that even with the best-coordinated and most effectively drilled emergency plans, there is no guarantee that what is expected to happen actually will happen. If the emergency is a broad disaster, such as an earthquake or a tornado, there is likely to be panic and chaos. This is why flexibility or the ability to improvise on-site is vital. The best disaster response is merely an extension of good daily emergency response but with the mobilization of larger numbers of personnel, supplies, and equipment.

In addition, for emergency planning to succeed it must be a coordinated effort between health care facility and community. With planning and practice, the facility can achieve a state of true preparedness that will enhance its response to, and recovery from, any type of emergency.

Environmental and Workplace Health

I n addition to the bloodborne pathogens, hazardous chemicals and wastes, and physical hazards discussed in earlier chapters, health care employees are exposed to a number of environmental hazards. For example, in some areas of the facility, employees may be exposed to patients with tuberculosis or other communicable diseases. Additionally, employees may be exposed to certain common chemicals that are known to cause reproductive health problems. However, by following appropriate guidelines and creating effective safety programs, employees can work safely in spite of these hazards.

This chapter identifies several environmental hazards that pose a threat to the health of employees in the health care facility. It also offers guidelines that have been developed to help facilities formulate programs to protect employees in the workplace.

☐ Tuberculosis

Tuberculosis (TB) is a recognized risk in health care facilities. In recent years, the increase in TB cases, including those involving multidrug-resistant strains, has heightened concern about facility transmission of the disease. In addition, in many areas the increase in TB cases is related to the high risk of TB among persons infected with human immunodeficiency virus (HIV). Transmission of TB is most likely to occur from patients who have unrecognized TB and who either are not on an effective therapy program or have not been placed in isolation.

To combat the spread of TB, the Centers for Disease Control and Prevention (CDC) has developed specific guidelines for health care facilities to follow. The guidelines state that an effective TB infection control plan should be based on taking certain control measures—administrative controls, engineering controls, and use of respirators.

Administrative controls involve development and implementation of written procedures to ensure early detection of persons with active TB and subsequent isolation. Isolation prevents or contains the spread of infectious airborne particles to caregivers and other parts of the facility.

Engineering controls prevent the spread of TB by reducing the amount of infectious material in the air. These controls include the following measures:

- Direct source control using local exhaust ventilation
- Airflow direction control to prevent contamination of air in areas adjacent to the infectious source
- Dilution and removal of contaminated air through the use of good ventilation engineering
- Air purification by use of air filtration or ultraviolet irradiation

Use of approved respirators reduces the risk of employee exposure to TB in areas where employees come into direct contact with TB patients. Respirators must be capable of removing TB bacteria completely. One type of respirator suitable for TB protection uses a HEPA filter.

In addition to these general control measures, the CDC has made a number of specific recommendations of safety elements that must be included as part of a sound TB program. These include the following:

- A risk assessment should be conducted for the facility as a whole and for individual areas where TB patients may receive care. (See figure 11-1 for a summary of elements in a risk assessment.)
- Responsibility for the design, implementation, and maintenance of the TB infection control program should be assigned to one individual.
- A written TB infection control program should be developed.
- Policies should be implemented to ensure early detection of patients who may have infectious TB.
- Prompt triage and appropriate management of outpatients who may have infectious TB should be provided.

Figure 11-1. Risk Assessment

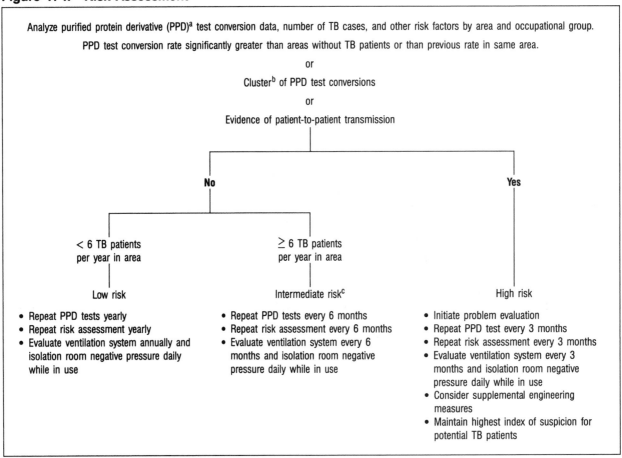

[a]PPD—Skin test

[b]Cluster = Two or more PPD conversions in one area or a single occupational group that works in multiple areas over a 3-month period

[c]Occurrence of drug-resistant TB in the facility or the community, or high prevalence of HIV infection among patients or workers in the facility may warrant a higher risk rating

Source: *Federal Register* 58(195), Oct. 12, 1993, 52816.

- Diagnostic evaluation, isolation, and treatment should be promptly initiated and maintained for persons who may have infectious TB and who are admitted to the inpatient setting.
- Ventilation and other engineering controls should be installed and maintained to reduce the potential for airborne exposure to TB.
- A respiratory protection program should be implemented.
- Appropriate precautions should be used for cough-inducing TB treatment procedures.
- Employees should be educated and trained in effective methods for prevention of TB transmission and in the benefits of medical screening programs.
- A routine employee TB screening program should be developed and implemented.
- Possible episodes of transmission of TB in health care facilities should be promptly evaluated, including positive TB skin test results, clusters of cases of TB in employees or patients, and contacts with TB patients who were not properly detected and isolated.
- Activities should be coordinated with the local public health department, emphasizing the reporting of TB cases and follow-up after discharge to ensure completion of therapy.

Figure 11-2 shows a TB control program recommended by the CDC.

☐ Respiratory Hazards

Respiratory hazards are not always easy to detect. Among the most common hazards are lack of oxygen and presence of harmful dust, fumes, gases, sprays, and disease-carrying organisms. Some of these hazards may cause cancer and other diseases. Certain types of respirators filter out and prevent entry of harmful substances into the lungs. Other types provide a separate supply of breathable air that is free of harmful material.

Engineering Controls

Usually, the use of respirators in health care facilities is limited to only a few employees. This is because the prevention of atmospheric contamination is accomplished as much as possible through engineering controls, including:

- Confining the material in a suitable enclosure
- Exhausting the material in an appropriate manner
- Substituting the material with a less hazardous material

Respirators are required when engineering controls are not yet in place or where controls are not completely effective. All personnel exposed to TB patients or other contaminated patients, hazardous material spills, or fire response situations should wear respirators.

Regulatory Requirements

When respirators are necessary, specific procedures must be followed to overcome potential equipment deficiencies and to ensure the effectiveness of the equipment. Employers are responsible for establishing an effective respiratory program in compliance with Occupational Safety and Health Administration (OSHA) regulations (OSHA 29 CFR 1910.134, Respiratory Protection Standard). Because of its technical nature, responsibility for the program should be assigned to someone trained in respiratory protection.

A respiratory program should stress thorough training of participants. Employees should be aware of the equipment's purpose and limitations, and should be instructed that the equipment must not be altered or removed during use, even for a short time. An effective respirator program includes the following requirements:

111

Figure 11-2. CDC TB Control Program for All Health Care Facilities

Table 1. Elements of the Risk Assessment

1. Review the number of TB patients seen, by area (inpatient and outpatient). (This information can be obtained by laboratory surveillance or medical record review.)
2. Review the drug-susceptibility patterns of TB patients seen at the facility.
3. Analyze HCW[a] PPD[b] test data, by area (or by occupational group for persons not assigned to a specific area such as respiratory therapists).

Review medical records of a sample of consecutive TB patients seen at the facility to evaluate infection control parameters.

Calculate intervals from

- Admission until TB suspected
- Admission until TB evaluation performed
- Admission until AFB specimens ordered
- AFB specimens ordered until AFB specimens collected
- AFB specimens collected until AFB smears done and reported
- AFB specimens collected until cultures done and reported
- AFB specimens collected until species identification done and reported
- AFB specimens collected until drug-susceptibility tests done and reported
- Admission until TB isolation initiated
- Admission until TB treatment initiated
- Duration of TB isolation

Additional Information

- Were appropriate criteria used for discontinuing isolation?
- History of prior admission to facility
- Adequacy of TB treatment regimen
- Were follow-up sputum specimens collected appropriately?
- Was appropriate discharge planning conducted?

Perform an observational review of TB infection control practices.

Perform a review of the most recent environmental evaluation and maintenance procedures.

Table 2. Optimum TB Control Program for All Health Care Facilities

I. Initial and Periodic Risk Assessment
   A. Evaluate HCW PPD test conversion data
   B. Determine TB prevalence among patients
   C. Reassess risk each PPD testing period
II. Written TB Infection Control Program
   A. Document all aspects of TB control
   B. Identify individual(s) responsible for TB control program
   C. Explain and emphasize hierarchy of controls
III. Implementation
   A. Assignment of Responsibility
      1. Assign responsibility for TB control program to individual(s)
      2. Ensure that persons with expertise in infection control, occupational health, and engineering are identified and included
   B. Risk Assessment and Periodic Reassessment of the Program
      1. Select initial risk protocols
      2. Observe HCW infection control practices
      3. Repeat risk assessment at appropriate intervals
   C. Early Detection of Patients With TB
      1. Symptom screen for each patient a. On initial encounter in ER or ambulatory care setting b. Before or at admission
      2. Radiologic and bacteriologic screening for patients with symptoms of TB
   D. Management of Outpatients with Possible Infectious TB
      1. Promptly initiate TB precautions
      2. Place patients in separate waiting areas of TB isolation rooms
      3. Give patients mask, box of tissues, instructions

Figure 11-2. (Continued)

E. Isolation for Infectious TB Patients
   1. Prompt isolation and initiation of treatment for patients with suspected or known infectious TB
   2. Monitoring of response to treatment
   3. Appropriate criteria for discontinuation of isolation
F. Engineering Recommendations
   1. Local exhaust and general ventilation should be designed in collaboration with persons with expertise in ventilation engineering
   2. In areas where infectious TB patients receive care, use single-pass system or recirculation after HEPA filtration
   3. Use additional measures, if needed, in areas where TB patients may receive care
   4. Health care facilities should be designed to achieve the best possible ventilation airflows
   5. Regularly monitor and maintain engineering controls
   6. Monitor and maintain TB isolation room negative pressure daily while in use relative to hallway and all surrounding areas
   7. Exhaust TB isolation room air to outside or, if unavoidable, recirculate after HEPA filtration
G. Respiratory Protection
   1. Respiratory protective devices should meet recommended performance criteria
   2. Should be worn by persons in settings where administrative and engineering controls are not likely to provide adequate protection (e.g., TB isolation rooms, treatment rooms, and other high-risk areas)
   3. A respiratory protection program is required where respiratory protection is used
H. Cough-Inducing Procedures
   1. Should not be performed on TB patients unless absolutely necessary
   2. Should be performed using local exhaust or in individual TB isolation room
   3. After completion, TB patients should remain in booth or enclosure until cough subsides
I. HCW TB Education
   1. All HCWs should receive periodic education appropriate to their job
   2. Should include epidemiology of TB in the facility
   3. Should emphasize concepts of pathogenesis and occupational risk
   4. Should describe practices that reduce TB transmission
J. HCW Counseling and Screening
   1. Counsel all HCWs regarding TB and TB infection
   2. Counsel all HCWs about increased risk if immunocompromised
   3. PPD test all HCWs on employment and repeat at periodic intervals
   4. Screen symptomatic HCWs for active TB
K. Evaluate HCW PPD Test Conversions and Possible Nosocomial TB Transmission
L. Coordinate Efforts with Public Health Department

[a]HCW—Health Care Worker

[b]PPD—Skin Test (Purified Protein Derivative)

Source: *Federal Register* 58(195), Oct. 12, 1993, 52817-52818.

- Employee use of the respirator should be in accordance with instructions and training received.
- Procedures governing the selection and use of the appropriate respirator should be in writing.
- Respirators should be selected on the basis of the hazards to which employees are exposed.
- Respirators used should be restricted to those approved by the Mine Safety and Health Administration and the National Institute for Occupational Safety and Health.
- Employees should be trained in the proper use and limitations of the specific respirator.
- Fit testing should be done to ensure proper protection.
- Instructions should be made available on proper respirator cleaning and disinfecting techniques.
- Respirators should be stored in a clean and sanitary location.
- Respirators should be inspected during cleaning and defective equipment replaced.
- Appropriate surveillance of workplace condition and degree of employee exposure or stress during respirator use should take place.
- The respirator program should be monitored and evaluated annually.

113

- Employees should undergo a medical examination to determine whether they are physically able to perform the work while using the respirator.
- Use of compressed gases supplied to respirators that meet applicable standards as described in OSHA regulations should be ensured.

When all the OSHA requirements for a respirator program are met, employees should be able to work in the presence of hazardous materials. However, the goal should always be to find a way to eliminate the need for respirators through the use of engineering controls.

☐ Ergonomic Hazards

Not all injuries occur as a result of a sudden event such as a fall or unexpected exposure to hazardous materials. Routine work, such as repetitive motion including the use of hands and arms, can also cause injury. When done improperly, repetitive lifting is often the cause of back injury. In recent years, there has been increased awareness of the many types of injuries caused by ergonomic hazards. *Ergonomics* is the science of managing the relationship between the individual and the work environment to prevent cumulative trauma disorders (CTDs), also referred to as repetitive strain disorders.

CTDs are a class of disorders involving damage to various parts of the body. Principally, the parts of the body affected are:

- Tendons
- Bones, muscles, and nerves of the hands and wrists
- Elbows
- Shoulders
- Neck and back

Because of increased concern over the number of CTDs reported industrywide, OSHA published a voluntary set of guidelines that recommend a framework for developing ergonomic safety programs. These guidelines include recommendations to assist employers in developing an effective mechanism to reduce CTDs. The recommendations provide a starting point for a program by focusing on the CTDs of the upper extremities and lower back disorders. The importance of management commitment and employee involvement is stressed and a program is recommended. Following are the program's major elements:

- Worksite analysis
- Hazard prevention and control
- Medical management
- Training and education

Worksite Analysis

The first step of a sound ergonomic program is to determine which jobs are sources of CTDs. This can be done by analyzing all medical and safety records for evidence of CTDs. Because CTDs often are recordable illnesses and injuries, the OSHA 200 log should be reviewed (see chapter 12 for an explanation of this form). Employee surveys and historical knowledge of high-risk jobs also can be used. If CTDs are found in significant numbers, an analysis should be made to identify trends or clusters.

The second step is to perform a more detailed analysis of jobs identified as causing, or having the potential to cause, CTDs. The purpose of this analysis is to identify the risk factors for CTDs in a specific job (see figure 11-3). Typical risk factors include:

- Excessive repetition
- Prolonged activity

Figure 11-3. Identifying Ergonomic At-Risk Task Sources

Workplace Characteristics

The following are some key factors which should be eliminated or minimized in every workplace or work method:

- Twisting, clothes-wringing motions of the wrist
- Working with a bent or flexed wrist
- Working with the neck bent at more that a 15° angle
- Vibration from power hand tools
- Using hand tools which are not balanced or which are difficult to hold
- Using hand tools that require a power grip force
- Using hand tools with a grip span of more than four inches between the thumb and forefinger
- Using hand tools with sharp edges or ridges
- Using hand tools that direct air exhaust onto the hand
- Repetitive hand, arm, and shoulder motions
- Holding the arms and elbows high or outstretched
- Working with controls, tools, or materials, which are beyond easy reach (beyond 14 inches)
- Working with controls that require too much force to operate
- Working with control systems that do not consider reflex actions in an emergency
- Working with the body leaning forward
- Repetitive manual handling
- Handling materials from heights above the shoulder or below the knee
- Excessive twisting or stretching
- Repetitive pushing or pulling, including requirements for high strength
- Standing or sitting for long periods
- Working in an immobile position for extended periods
- Static muscular work (requires maintenance of unsupported muscles during work task)
- Working in an environment with a lack of adjustable work surfaces or chairs
- Sitting on poorly designed chairs

Reprinted, with permission, from *Baxter Ergonomic Guidelines.* Deerfield, IL: Baxter Health Care Corporation, 1993.

- Forceful exertion with the hands
- Awkward posture of the body
- Improper seating and back support

Hazard Prevention and Control

Once a job has been identified as presenting ergonomic hazards, preventive measures can be taken. Ergonomic hazards are prevented primarily by an effective redesign of the job or job site. This involves the use of appropriate engineering, work practice, and administrative controls.

Engineering controls are the preferred methods of control. The primary focus of engineering controls is to make the job fit the person, rather than force the person to fit the demands of the job. This can be accomplished by redesigning the workstation, work methods, work tools, and/or work requirements. The purpose of the redesign is to reduce or eliminate excessive exertion, repetitive motion, awkward postures, and other risk factors.

Administrative controls also can reduce employee exposure to tasks with ergonomic hazards. For example, employee exposure could be reduced through rotation to less stressful jobs, reduced workloads and rest, exercise, or stretching breaks.

Medical Management

A medical program is essential to the success of a total ergonomic program. As with other injuries or illnesses, employees should be encouraged to inform their supervisor if they experience discomfort or other symptoms that may be caused by CTDs. The supervisor should have the employee see a physician as soon as possible and should document the employee's concern. Prompt medical attention will allow the physician to determine if the problem is a CTD and to recommend appropriate action before the condition becomes more serious. Physicians

115

involved in treating CTDs should have training in the prevention, early recognition, treatment, and rehabilitation of CTD disorders. Supervisors should be aware that some CTD injuries are OSHA reportable and should follow up on each suspected case. Proper use of reporting and medical attention can keep CTDs from becoming serious disabilities that could lead to employee suffering, lost time, and workers' compensation claims.

Training and Education

Perhaps the most important element of an effective ergonomic program is training and education. The purpose of training and education is to ensure that employees are sufficiently informed about CTD risks to which they may be exposed, thereby allowing them to participate actively in their own protection. A training program should involve all affected employees, engineers and maintenance personnel, and supervisors and managers.

The training program should be designed and implemented by qualified personnel, and appropriate special training should be provided for those responsible for administering the program. The program should be presented at a level of understanding appropriate for the individuals being trained. It should provide an overview of the potential risk of illnesses and injuries, their causes and early symptoms, means of prevention, and treatment.

The training program also should include a means for adequately evaluating its effectiveness. This can be achieved by using employee interviews, testing employees, and observing work practices to determine whether those who received the training understand the material and the work practice to be followed.

☐ Reproductive Health Hazards

Exposure to certain agents in health care facilities presents reproductive hazards to employees of child-bearing age, as well as to the fetus. Following are some of the adverse problems that can result from exposure to these agents:

- Birth defects
- Infertility
- Impotence
- Spontaneous abortion
- Increased infant mortality
- Childhood cancer

Identifying Hazardous Agents

Some of the agents that can cause reproductive problems are many chemicals commonly used in health care facilities. For example:

- Anesthetic gases used in surgery can reduce female fertility and cause spontaneous abortion.
- Ethylene oxide (EtO) used to sterilize equipment can cause spontaneous abortion.
- Mercury used in laboratories can cause menstrual disorders and spontaneous abortion.
- Lead used in X-ray procedures can cause premature birth and spontaneous abortion. It also can cause decreased sperm count in males.
- Xylene used in laboratories can cause menstrual disorders.

Biological hazards that adversely affect reproduction include a number of infectious agents. For example:

- Syphilis
- Rubella (mumps)

- German measles
- Herpes simplex
- Hepatitis
- Chicken pox
- HIV

In addition to chemical and biological hazards, ionizing radiation from X rays and nuclear medicines pose reproductive and fetal risks. Radiation also can cause decreased sperm count in men.

Developing a Reproductive Health Policy

Developing a reproductive management policy involves implementation of program elements similar to those used in the management of bloodborne pathogens and other hazardous substances. The first step is to perform a risk assessment to identify the location and the employee exposure potential for all chemical and biological reproductive hazards. The next step is to develop and implement a policy that will require the following:

- Universal precautions for biological hazards
- Monitoring of work areas to minimize chemical exposure
- Educating employees about reproductive risks
- Training employees in the proper procedures and protective measures
- Providing and enforcing the use of personal protective equipment
- Providing medical surveillance for all employees accidentally exposed through routine job tasks
- Investigating all exposure incidents and taking corrective action
- Upgrading the program as new information becomes available

As research into the hazards of chemicals progresses, many more substances are being linked to harmful effects on the reproductive system. These effects may require years—even generations—to appear. A process must be in place to evaluate new reproductive hazards information and implement procedures to protect employees from the effects of reproductive health hazards.

□ Conclusion

Health care workers are exposed to many types of hazards that can cause injury and health problems. Protection against these hazards requires strict implementation of preventive measures and protective equipment. Tuberculosis, cumulative trauma disorders, and reproductive health hazards are examples of hazards that health care workers face every day. However, the process for managing these hazards is feasible and involves conducting a risk assessment to define the problem, developing procedures, and training employees. Once these elements are in place, employees can work safely while carrying out their job assignments.

Incident Reporting and Investigation

A comprehensive safety program is of prime importance in minimizing the occurrence of safety-related incidents. However, even with implementation of an effective safety program, a facility cannot always prevent incidents from occurring. When incidents do occur, it is the health care facility's responsibility to observe proper follow-up procedures, which should include determining the cause of the incident and taking corrective measures.

Additionally, it is important that the facility develop a recordkeeping system for incidents, as well as guidelines for determining which incidents are serious enough to warrant further examination. This can be accomplished through a standardized system for incident reporting and investigation.

Proper reporting of all incidents helps management review situations and make corrections to prevent potential injury. It also develops a historical record for management to observe and analyze for possible recurrent situations. By following a standardized system for incident reporting, facilities can avoid injuries, minimize property damage, and save lives.

This chapter discusses the principal elements involved in incident reporting. It also describes various techniques that can be used in the investigation of incidents.

☐ Incident Reporting

The term *incident* generally is defined as an unexpected, undesired happening that has the potential to adversely affect the completion of a task or to cause injury or property damage. The following subsections describe what incidents in the health care facility should be reported, who should fill out incident reports, what information should be included, and how reports should be routed.

What Incidents Should Be Reported

First, all incidents should be reported; and, second, all incidents should be reported in a standard format. The policy of many facilities is to report only the more severe injuries or accidents; however, because less serious incidents often predict the occurrence of more damaging events, this approach to incident reporting often is a mistake. Incidents that could be classified as "near misses" should signal staff that a situation exists which may cause an accident to occur. For example, should a visitor complain at a nurses' station that she slipped on a slick spot on the restroom floor, her complaint should be addressed immediately. Although no injury or property damage occurred, the complaint signals that the potential for injury exists. An incident report should be completed and then given to the risk manager or safety director. As part of the data-tracking system, the risk manager or safety director should also record the action taken. These actions attest to the facility's concern for safety and willingness to improve hazardous conditions.

Prompt reporting of all incidents provides documentation of the measures the employer takes to protect the health and life of facility employees, patients, visitors, and volunteers. Additionally, this documentation may be necessary as evidence in several situations, such as Joint Commission on Accreditation of Healthcare Organizations (JCAHO) reviews, workers' compensation procedures, state and local agency inspections, and during inspections by the Occupational Safety and Health Administration (OSHA). For these reasons, all incidents should be reported, whether or not injury or property damage resulted.

Another frequent and costly mistake in health care incident reporting occurs when only safety-related incidents, such as falls or accidental injuries, are reported. Adverse outcomes of clinical care and actions during that care are sometimes excluded from the incident-reporting procedure. This amounts to a risky oversight and one that could be expensive for the facility, because clinical incidents are most likely to result in malpractice claims against both caregiver and facility.

Although documenting clinical incidents, often called *occurrence reporting*, typically is a quality assurance function, the safety department or the safety director should work with quality assurance personnel to devise a coordinated system if none currently exists. This liaison should be ongoing, because clinical treatment and patient, employee, and visitor activities ancillary to patient care regularly intersect and have an impact on one another.

Who Should Report the Incident

To some extent, the reporting system depends on the facility's routine. Some organizations require supervisors to report the incidents in which their employees are involved. Although this system encourages the involvement and concern of supervisors, it has several drawbacks. For instance, it removes employees from a process that directly affects them. In addition, having the supervisor fill out the incident report may give it the appearance of a disciplinary action and the employee may become reluctant to tell the whole story.

The best person to describe exactly what happened is the employee involved in the incident. Whenever possible, employees should complete their own incident reports or at least be involved in the process. This gives them a sense of control over how the incident is viewed by management. It also eliminates the inaccuracies associated with communicating a story through a chain of people. Additionally, employee incident reporting can be an excellent way to involve employees in safety. As employees participate more fully in safety, they will begin to embrace the safety program's goals as their own.

The incident-reporting system should require the supervisor to review the incident and, when possible, discuss it with the employee. In this way, both supervisory and line employee involvement are maintained. (See figure 12-1 for a flowchart of supervisory actions in response to employee injuries.)

To ensure regular and appropriate reporting by all staff members, the facility must provide training and education in incident-reporting techniques. All employees should receive training in when to file a report, how to fill it out, and whom to send it to. (See chapter 13 for a discussion of training methods.)

During training, the benefits to the employee of incident reporting should be specified, namely, that the reports will be used to reduce hazards and prevent future incidents. It also should be emphasized that in most circumstances, the reports will not be used against employees in any disciplinary action. Management should assure employees that action will be taken to prevent further incidents. It is important to emphasize that managers should be true to their word. Nothing motivates employees to participate in incident reporting more than the knowledge that their reports will get results.

Figure 12-1. Flowchart: Action Plan for Response to Employee Injuries

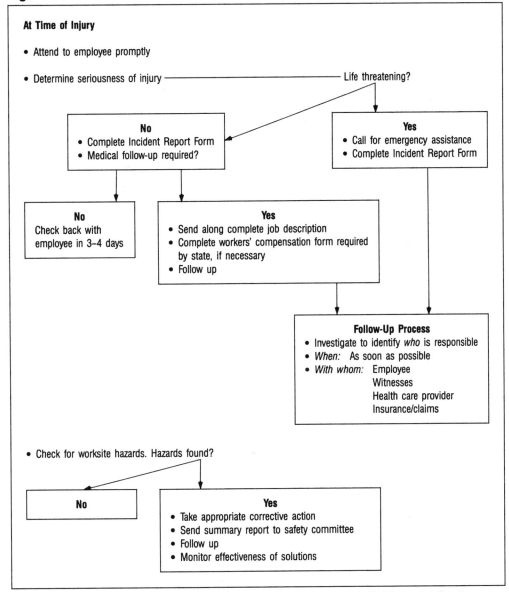

Adapted, with permission, from *Case Management of Employee Incidents*, published by Fred S. James & Co. of Minnesota, Inc., 1986.

What Information Should Be Reported

There probably are as many incident report forms as there are facilities to report incidents. No one form can truly be considered ideal for every facility; to a large extent, the form used depends on the methods, style, needs, and preferences of the individual facility. However, there are some basic types of forms and some basic questions that all forms should ask.

Two major types of forms have emerged—the traditional narrative format and the checklist approach. The narrative format (figure 12-2) gives the writer more space to answer questions and to elaborate on and personalize the occurrence.

In the checklist approach (figure 12-3), incidents are divided into categories (for example, "fall" or "patient complaint") and the appropriate box is checked. Using a computer program allows the computer to determine trends in types of incidents, times of day, shifts, and characteristics of personnel involved. Both forms have their virtues, although the trend is toward forms

121

Figure 12-2. Sample Incident Report: Narrative Format

cc Administration
Dept. Head
Safety Committee

James

SUPERVISOR'S REPORT OF EMPLOYEE INCIDENT

CLAIM NO. _____

NOTE: This report is to be promptly and fully completed by employee's supervisor or designee except where noted. A response to all questions is required unless otherwise indicated.

Date of Incident _____
Date Supv. Notified _____
Date Report Completed _____

_____ Near Miss   _____ Medical Follow-up

_____ First Aid   _____ Property Damage

WHO

Name _____ Age _____ Sex _____

Soc. Sec. No. _____ Position _____ Dept. _____

Full/Part time (Circle)   Permanent/Temporary (Circle)

Was employee engaged in usual work when incident occurred? (If not, specify position and date assigned): _____
_____

Names of other individuals involved: _____

Witnesses: _____

WHEN

Time _____ AM/PM   Day: S M T W TH F SA   Shift: First Second Third

WHERE

Location (identify precisely): _____
_____

HOW

Incident description (include specific description of employee's activities at time of incident): _____
_____
_____
_____

Identify physical/mechanical objects involved (tools, supplies, equipment, structures, etc. List mfg., model, and serial no.): _____
_____

Pre-existing disability/condition contributing to incident? (specify): _____

Back Injuries ONLY: Were appropriate transfer techniques/lifting assists (transfer belt, patient lift, etc.) being utilized? (If YES, specify device): _____

INCIDENT CAUSES (Check all that apply):

EQUIPMENT:
_____ Inappropriate for task
_____ Inadequate maintenance
_____ Inadequate design
_____ Other (MUST specify): _____

PERSONAL:
_____ Failure to comply with established policies/procedures
_____ Failure to use appropriate equipment/techniques
_____ Lack of familiarity with task
_____ Improper motivation/attitude
_____ Other (MUST specify): _____

ENVIRONMENTAL:
_____ Wet Surface
_____ Inadequate guards
_____ Fire hazard
_____ Congestion
_____ Electrical hazard
_____ Other (MUST specify): _____

PROCEDURAL:
_____ Inadequate specification of equipment standards
_____ Inadequate specification of policies/procedures
_____ Inadequate communication of policies/procedures
_____ Inadequate enforcement of policies/procedures
_____ Other (MUST specify): _____

Form 86-1 Rev. 9/86

Figure 12-2. (Continued)

WHAT	Describe nature and severity of injuries or property damage: _____ _____ _____ INCIDENT TYPES (Check all that apply): ____ Unexpected movement/sprain/strain ____ Chemical irritant ____ Struck by object/person ____ Fall from elevation ____ Puncture ____ Struck against object ____ Fall on level ____ Laceration ____ Caught between objects ____ Motor vehicle ____ Burn ____ Other (specify): _____
LOSS PREVENTION	Will employee lose work time as a result of the above? _____ What recommendations do you have to prevent a reoccurrence of this type of incident? _____ _____ _____ What actions are you taking or intend to take to prevent a reoccurrence of this type of incident? _____ _____ _____ Employee referred to: ____ Agency Clinic ____ EMS ____ Personal MD ____ Other (specify): _____
EMPLOYEE REVIEW	Above reviewed with employee; employee comments: _____ _____ _____ _____ _____ _____ _____ Employee Signature/Date Supervisor Signature/Date
DEPARTMENT REVIEW	Does this work area have previous history of incidents? (If YES, indicate date of most recent incident and number of incidents in past 12 months): _____ Has above physical/mechanical object been involved in a previous incident? (If YES, indicate most recent incident and number of incidents in past 12 months): _____ Does this employee have previous history of incidents? (If YES, indicate date of most recent incident and number of incidents in the past 12 months): _____ Date employee hired: _____ Date filled current position: _____ Department Head comments: _____ _____ _____ _____ Date First Report of Injury completed: _____ Date First Report forwarded to James: _____ _____ Department Head Signature/Date
ADMINISTRATIVE REVIEW	Administration Comments: _____ _____ _____ _____ _____ _____ _____ Signature/Date

Reprinted, with permission, from Fred. S. James & Co. of Minnesota, Inc., 1986.

Figure 12-3. Sample Incident Report: Checklist Format

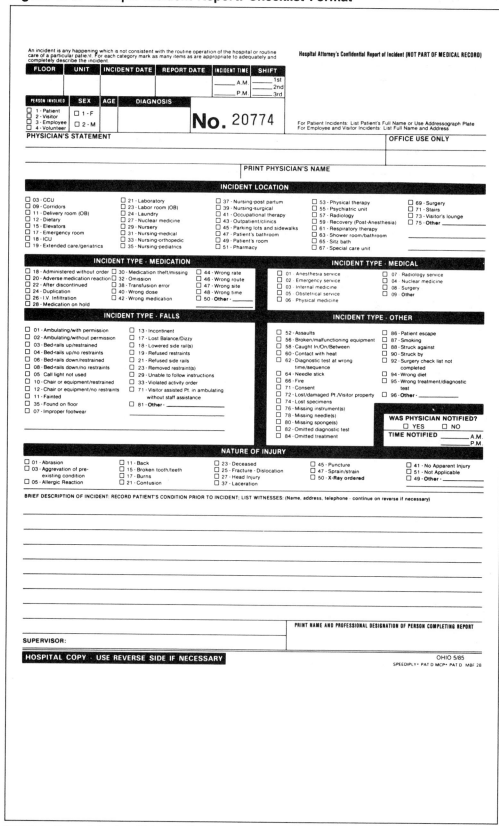

Reprinted, with permission, from Wade, R. D. *Risk Management—HPL, Hospital Professional Liability Primer*. Columbus, OH: Ohio Insurance Company, 1981, pp. 88–89.

that are amenable to computer analysis. Checklists are acceptable as long as they provide room for narrative and difficult-to-classify incidents, and generally balance categorization with explanation.

Whatever form is selected, it should be short (no longer than the front and back of one page), should use questions that are easily understood, and should be as concise as possible while still eliciting the necessary facts. Some of the more important information to be obtained from any incident report form could be elicited by the following questions:

- *Who was involved in the incident?* This includes the individual's full name and age and whether he or she is a patient, employee, volunteer, or visitor. If the person is an employee, his or her job title, department, and hire date also should be noted.
- *Where did the incident occur?* This request is for the exact location and should be answered as precisely as possible. For example, an answer of "east hallway outside room 516" or "east hallway, 10 feet from nurses' station" is preferable to "5th floor corridor."
- *When did the incident occur?* This answer should include the date, day of the week, exact time, and shift. This specific information aids in determining whether time of day, shift, and so on increase the likelihood of this type of incident.
- *What kind of incident occurred?* Either the appropriate box should be checked or the occurrence should be categorized (for example, medication error, hazardous condition, theft, and so on).
- *Were there any injuries, and what type of damage, if any, resulted from the incident?* Any injuries should be described, and it should be noted whether a physician was notified. Any property damage also should be described.
- *How did the incident occur?* This is where a concise but informative narrative is required. Events leading up to the incident should be detailed, and any equipment or machinery involved should be listed, including name of manufacturer, model number, and serial number. Also, the work being performed at the time of the incident should be explained.
- *Why did the incident occur?* This is an important question, but one that can create many problems. The information should state the contributing factors and causes of the incident, not the blame. Incidents are rarely the result of a single cause, although one cause may be more obvious than another. For example, in the case of an employee suffering injury from a fall off a ladder, the accident investigation report may state that the ladder was defective. In order to locate and define additional contributing factors and causes, other questions must be asked. For example:
  —Why was the defective ladder available for use?
  —Why was the ladder defective?
  —Why didn't the injured person know not to use the ladder?
  —Are there other ladders in the facility like this one?
  —Has this happened before?
  Objectivity in determining the incident's true cause is crucial. The supervisor should assist the employee in discovering the causes. If management system deficiencies contributed to the incident, they should be clearly identified and corrected. It is defeating to pass all incidents off merely as results of employee carelessness or willful negligence. Instead of claiming the employee was careless, an effort should be made to find out if he or she knew what to do, followed instructions, used safe work methods, had the necessary skills, received proper training, and so on.
- *What measures can be taken to correct these problems or remove factors that cause incidents?* Having those involved recommend actions to be taken may provide excellent ideas that supervisors may not have considered. However, not all incident reports ask for this information. Instead, corrective actions sometimes are elicited on separate follow-up forms.

After the incident report form is completed, it should be signed and dated.

How the Report Should Be Routed

The chain of people through which the incident report is routed should be kept to a minimum. In this way, confidentiality is maintained and, equally important, action is not delayed while the report is being reviewed. The first person to receive the report should be the employee's immediate supervisor, who assists the employee in completing the form.

In most cases, the incident report is passed on, preferably within 24 hours, to the safety director, risk manager, or other designated individual. This person reviews the incident and determines whether an investigation is necessary. The safety director or risk manager also decides whether anyone else needs to see the report, such as the administrator or chief executive officer, employee health personnel, insurance representatives, the safety committee, or legal counsel. The number of persons within the facility who see the report should be limited. Distributing the report to numerous departments or individuals not only violates confidentiality and discourages future reporting, but also may fragment follow-up efforts. Photocopies of the report should be made at the discretion of the safety director or risk manager only.

☐ OSHA Reporting

Health care facilities fall within the Standard Industrial Code (SIC) under OSHA recordkeeping requirements. Data from these records are used to compile factual information about accidents that have happened, to provide employers with a measure for evaluating the success of their safety programs, and to identify high-risk areas to which attention should be directed. OSHA reporting is separate and distinct from any insurance or workers' compensation documentation. The major requirements focus on two forms: OSHA Form 200 and OSHA Form 101.

Form 200, called the Log and Summary of Occupational Injuries and Illnesses, is used by organizations to compile their injury and illness statistics for each calendar year. It categorizes the incidents and furnishes room for detailed analysis. A copy of the totals and other specific information must be posted in the facility where such notices are customarily posted, from February 1 to March 1 of the following year.

Form 101 documents each *recordable* (a term defined in OSHA regulations) illness or injury. In this case, the facility's incident report form may be acceptable, assuming it documents at least the facts requested on Form 101. The information gathered on the facility's form must be maintained for at least five years.

☐ Medical Device and Product Reporting

As discussed in chapter 2, the Food and Drug Administration (FDA) requires mandatory reporting under the Safe Medical Device Act (SMDA). In addition, the FDA has implemented a voluntary reporting program called MEDWatch, which is discussed later in this chapter.

SMDA Reporting Requirements

The Safe Medical Device Act (SMDA) of 1990 requires health care facilities to report information that reasonably suggests that a device has or may have caused or contributed to the death, serious illness, or injury of a patient. A *device* is defined as anything that is used in treatment or diagnosis, other than drugs. Examples include:

- X-ray machine
- Suture
- Defibrillator
- Vascular graft
- Syringe
- Surgical laser

- Heating pad
- Bone screw
- Gauze pad
- Patient restraint
- Infusion pump
- Hospital bed

Reports of death must be made to the FDA and the manufacturer of the device, if known. Reports of serious illness or injury must be made to the manufacturer or to the FDA if the manufacturer is unknown.

Device-related problems often are discovered by hospital personnel who use or maintain the devices, or by personnel conducting chart reviews. Such problems should be reported in accordance with the facilitywide program and analyzed to determine whether an SMDA user report (figure 12-4) must be submitted to the manufacturer and/or the FDA.

To meet SMDA requirements, every device-related problem must be reported and analyzed to determine whether reporting is required. A reporting flowchart (figure 12-5) may be helpful to include in the facility's policies and procedures relating to medical device reporting.

MEDWatch Reporting

MEDWatch is the FDA's name for its medical products reporting program. It is a broad program encompassing voluntary and mandatory reporting for medical products, including:

- Drugs
- Medical devices
- Biologicals
- Nutritional products

The FDA has developed two separate reporting forms. Form 3500 (figure 12-6, p. 131) is the FDA's *voluntary* report form, meaning that its submission is not mandated by law or regulation. This form is to be used to report serious adverse events associated with drugs, biologics, medical devices, nutritional products, or other FDA-regulated products. The form is submitted directly to the FDA, not to the manufacturer. Reports are encouraged if one of the products was associated with a serious outcome (such as death), a life-threatening condition, initial or prolonged hospitalization, a disability, a congenital anomaly, or a condition that required surgical or medical intervention to prevent permanent impairment or damage. Reports of product quality problems such as device defects, inaccurate or unreadable product labeling, packaging or product mix-up, contamination or stability problems, and particulate matter in injectable products also are encouraged.

Form 3500A (figure 12-7, p. 132) is a multipurpose form used for *mandatory* reporting of medical devices in accordance with SMDA. It must be used by user facilities, distributors, and manufacturers. The form also is to be used by manufacturers of drugs and biologics that are or will be required to submit medication-related adverse event reports to the FDA.

The goals of MEDWatch are to encourage reporting of adverse events so that appropriate responses can be taken. MEDWatch voluntary forms can be collected by the facility as a source of risk management/quality assurance information. This also may help to identify events that must be reported under SMDA, to centralize facilitywide event reporting, and to identify any conflicting reports. A centralized internal system also will help identify duplicate reports submitted by health professionals. Duplicate reports are likely because the criteria for submitting a device-related voluntary report are identical to those for mandatory SMDA reports.

☐ Techniques for Incident Investigation

The facility's safety department or safety committee should have established criteria to assist in determining which incidents require investigation. Safety staff should be familiar with

Figure 12-4. Medical Device Incident Investigation Form

Medical Device Incident Investigation Form

CONFIDENTIAL — FOR INTERNAL RISK MANAGEMENT PURPOSES ONLY

DO NOT PHOTOCOPY OR FILE IN MEDICAL RECORD

Case Identifier No. _____

I. DEVICE INFORMATION

Record for each device involved in incident, including disposables. Use separate forms as necessary.

Manufacturer name _____

_____

Brand name _____

_____

Generic product name _____

_____

Model number _____

Catalog number _____

Serial number _____

Lot number _____

Internal equipment control
   number_____

Expiration date _____

Purchase date _____

Labeled for single use? _____

Previously used?_____

Implanted device? _____

   Implantation date _____

Reusable device? _____

Cleaning/sterilization method
   used _____

_____

Collect the following: purchase contract, package insert, user/operator manual, maintenance contracts, recall notices.

II. SERVICE INFORMATION

Last date serviced _____

Service performed by_____

Was service on schedule? _____

Attach service records.

III. EVENT INFORMATION

Event result (death, injury, illness,
   malfunction) _____

Date of event _____

Specific injury incurred _____

Date that medical personnel became
   aware of the event _____

Date reported to
   manufacturer _____

Was device used as labeled/intended?
   (attach copy of label) _____

Device operator when event occurred
   (name, title) _____

_____

Location of event _____

Other relevant devices in use at time of
   event _____

_____

_____

_____

_____

Brief event description (what
   happened, how was device
   involved). Attach expanded
   narrative if needed. _____

_____

_____

_____

_____

_____

_____

_____

_____

Witnesses to event (name, title, phone)

_____

_____

_____

_____

_____

_____

_____

_____

_____

_____

IV. PATIENT INFORMATION

Record for each patient involved. Use separate forms as necessary.

Name _____

Address _____

_____

Phone _____

Classification (inpatient, outpatient,
   visitor, employee)_____

Patient ID no. _____

Room number _____

Age ____ Sex ____ Weight _____

Attending physician _____

_____

Known allergies _____

Diagnosis before event _____

Medical status before event
   (e.g., stable, critical, fair) _____
Was more than one patient
   involved?_____

If so, collect information for all
   patients.

Figure 12-4. **(Continued)**

V. *INJURY ASSESSMENT*

Time of discovery _____

Elapsed time from placement of
device _____

Description of injury _____

_____

_____

Location of injury on patient (e.g., head)

_____

Location of suspect device in relation to
injury _____

Extent of injury at time of discovery

_____

_____

Were photos of injury taken? (if yes,
attach to this form) _____

Patient treatment _____

_____

_____

Patient follow-up (current status)

_____

_____

VI. *INCIDENT INVESTIGATION*

*Collect relevant data for each device
involved in incident, including disposables. Use separate forms as necessary.*

Date reported to risk management

_____

Date investigation initiated _____

Switch/control/indicator settings at
time of incident (indicate whether
typical—y or n) _____

_____

_____

_____

_____

_____

Relevant environmental conditions

_____

_____

Has device malfunctioned before?

_____

When? _____

Description of prior malfunction

_____

Was report filed? _____

Was corrective action taken or repair
performed? (describe) _____

_____

_____

Positions and conditions of device,
accessories, disposables _____

_____

_____

_____

_____

_____

On a separate sheet, sketch
positions relative to patient.

Who inspected the device following
incident? _____

Did the device manufacturer witness the
inspection? _____

Name of witness _____

_____

Types of tests performed
(e.g.,electrical) _____

Inspection findings (Did device fail?
How? What components, attached
devices, or subassemblies failed?
Was the device used correctly?)
Attach expanded narrative if
needed.

_____

_____

_____

_____

_____

_____

VII. *INVESTIGATION CONCLUSIONS*

Was the device the direct cause of
the event? _____

How did the device cause or
contribute to the event? _____

_____

_____

_____

_____

_____

_____

_____

_____

_____

Immediate actions required

_____

_____

_____

_____

_____

_____

_____

Follow-up required

_____

_____

_____

_____

_____

_____

_____

_____

Figure 12-5. User Reporting Program

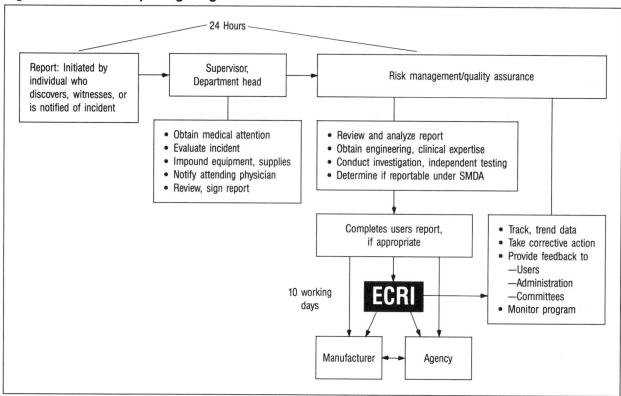

©1991 ECRI. Reprinted, with permission, from *Medical Device Reporting Under the Safe Medical Devices Act: A Guide for Healthcare Facilities.*

investigative techniques and principles. The safety office must be well organized with the facilities and have the capacity not only to conduct precautionary or initial investigations, but also to store and preserve investigative data and reports for use and reference at a later time should the incidents mature into claim or suit status. There are two types of investigation—informal and formal.

Informal Investigation

An informal investigation can be accomplished quickly and easily by the supervisor while working with the employee to complete the incident report. This type of investigation consists of an overview of the scene and a brief discussion with the employee and other persons involved. This can be done for every incident. The supervisor briefly notes the result of the investigation on a separate sheet, which is signed, dated, and forwarded with the report.

Formal Investigation

When an in-depth inquiry is necessary, the safety director, risk manager or supervisor, and safety staff conduct a formal investigation. Knowing which incidents warrant investigation is a skill that can be developed with practice. It is not always true that only incidents resulting in severe injury or property damage should be investigated. Some near-miss incidents may suggest serious hazards that could cause a major accident and thus should be investigated. In general, conditions that suggest the need for formal investigation include:

- Fatalities
- Patient or employee injuries
- A number of similar patient, employee, or visitor complaints
- A trend in time, place, or person involved in incidents
- A pattern of mishaps related to particular equipment or machinery

Figure 12-6. MEDWatch Reporting Form—Voluntary

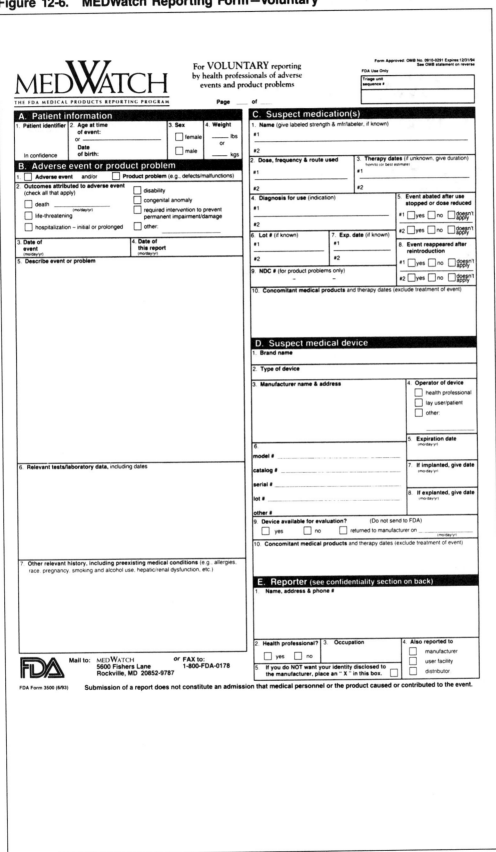

Figure 12-7. MEDWatch Reporting Form—Mandatory

MEDWATCH

THE FDA MEDICAL PRODUCTS REPORTING PROGRAM

For use by user-facilities, distributors and manufacturers for MANDATORY reporting

Page ___ of ___

Form Approved: OMB No. 0910-0291 Expires: 12/31/94
See OMB statement on reverse

Mfr report #

UF/Dist report #

FDA Use Only

A. Patient information

1. Patient identifier — In confidence
2. Age at time of event: or Date of birth:
3. Sex — ☐ female ☐ male
4. Weight — ___ lbs or ___ kgs

B. Adverse event or product problem

1. ☐ Adverse event and/or ☐ Product problem (e.g., defects/malfunctions)
2. Outcomes attributed to adverse event (check all that apply)
   - ☐ death ___ (mo/day/yr)
   - ☐ life-threatening
   - ☐ hospitalization – initial or prolonged
   - ☐ disability
   - ☐ congenital anomaly
   - ☐ required intervention to prevent permanent impairment/damage
   - ☐ other: ___
3. Date of event (mo/day/yr)
4. Date of this report (mo/day/yr)
5. Describe event or problem
6. Relevant tests/laboratory data, including dates
7. Other relevant history, including preexisting medical conditions (e.g., allergies, race, pregnancy, smoking and alcohol use, hepatic/renal dysfunction, etc.)

C. Suspect medication(s)

1. Name (give labeled strength & mfr/labeler, if known) — #1 / #2
2. Dose, frequency & route used — #1 / #2
3. Therapy dates (if unknown, give duration) from/to (or best estimate) — #1 / #2
4. Diagnosis for use (indication) — #1 / #2
5. Event abated after use stopped or dose reduced — #1 ☐ yes ☐ no ☐ doesn't apply; #2 ☐ yes ☐ no ☐ doesn't apply
6. Lot # (if known) — #1 / #2
7. Exp. date (if known) — #1 / #2
8. Event reappeared after reintroduction — #1 ☐ yes ☐ no ☐ doesn't apply; #2 ☐ yes ☐ no ☐ doesn't apply
9. NDC # – for product problems only (if known) — ___ - ___ - ___
10. Concomitant medical products and therapy dates (exclude treatment of event)

D. Suspect medical device

1. Brand name
2. Type of device
3. Manufacturer name & address
4. Operator of device — ☐ health professional ☐ lay user/patient ☐ other: ___
5. Expiration date (mo/day/yr)
6. model # ___ catalog # ___ serial # ___ lot # ___ other # ___
7. If implanted, give date (mo/day/yr)
8. If explanted, give date (mo/day/yr)
9. Device available for evaluation? (Do not send to FDA) ☐ yes ☐ no ☐ returned to manufacturer on ___ (mo/day/yr)
10. Concomitant medical products and therapy dates (exclude treatment of event)

E. Initial reporter

1. Name, address & phone #
2. Health professional? ☐ yes ☐ no
3. Occupation
4. Initial reporter also sent report to FDA ☐ yes ☐ no ☐ unk

FDA

FDA Form 3500A (6/93)

Submission of a report does not constitute an admission that medical personnel, user facility, distributor, manufacturer or product caused or contributed to the event.

Figure 12-7. (Continued)

Medication and Device Experience Report
(continued)
Refer to guidelines for specific instructions

Submission of a report does not constitute an admission that medical personnel, user facility, distributor, manufacturer or product caused or contributed to the event.

U.S. DEPARTMENT OF HEALTH AND HUMAN SERVICES
Public Health Service • Food and Drug Administration

Page ____ of ____

FDA Use Only

F. For use by user facility/distributor–devices only

1. Check one
☐ user facility ☐ distributor

2. UF/Dist report number

3. User facility or distributor name/address

4. Contact person

5. Phone Number

6. Date user facility or distributor became aware of event (mo/day/yr)

7. Type of report
☐ initial
☐ follow-up # ____

8. Date of this report (mo/day/yr)

9. Approximate age of device

10. Event problem codes (refer to coding manual)
patient code ____ – ____ – ____
device code ____ – ____ – ____

11. Report sent to FDA?
☐ yes ____ (mo/day/yr)
☐ no

12. Location where event occurred
☐ hospital
☐ home
☐ nursing home
☐ outpatient treatment facility
☐ other: ____
specify
☐ outpatient diagnostic facility
☐ ambulatory surgical facility

13. Report sent to manufacturer?
☐ yes ____ (mo/day/yr)
☐ no

14. Manufacturer name/address

G. All manufacturers

1. Contact office – name/address (& mfring site for devices)

2. Phone number

3. Report source (check all that apply)
☐ foreign
☐ study
☐ literature
☐ consumer
☐ health professional
☐ user facility
☐ company representative
☐ distributor
☐ other:

4. Date received by manufacturer (mo/day/yr)

5. (A)NDA # ____
IND # ____
PLA # ____
pre-1938 ☐ yes
OTC product ☐ yes

6. If IND, protocol #

7. Type of report (check all that apply)
☐ 5-day ☐ 15-day
☐ 10-day ☐ periodic
☐ initial ☐ follow-up # ____

8. Adverse event term(s)

9. Mfr. report number

H. Device manufacturers only

1. Type of reportable event
☐ death
☐ serious injury
☐ malfunction (see guidelines)
☐ other: ____

2. If follow-up, what type?
☐ correction
☐ additional information
☐ response to FDA request
☐ device evaluation

3. Device evaluated by mfr?
☐ not returned to mfr.
☐ yes ☐ evaluation summary attached
☐ no (attach page to explain why not) or provide code: ____

4. Device manufacture date (mo/yr)

5. Labeled for single use?
☐ yes ☐ no

6. Evaluation codes (refer to coding manual)
method ____ – ____ – ____
results ____ – ____ – ____
conclusions ____ – ____ – ____

7. If remedial action initiated, check type
☐ recall ☐ notification
☐ repair ☐ inspection
☐ replace ☐ patient monitoring
☐ relabeling ☐ modification/ adjustment
☐ other:

8. Usage of device
☐ initial use of device
☐ reuse
☐ unknown

9. If action reported to FDA under 21 USC 360i(f), list correction/removal reporting number:

10. ☐ Additional manufacturer narrative and/or 11. ☐ Corrected data

The public reporting burden for this collection of information has been estimated to average one-hour per response, including the time for reviewing instructions, searching existing data sources, gathering and maintaining the data needed, and completing and reviewing the collection of information. Send your comments regarding this burden estimate or any other aspect of this collection of information, including suggestions for reducing this burden to:

Reports Clearance Officer, PHS
Hubert H. Humphrey Building, Room 721-B
200 Independance Avenue, S.W.
Washington, DC 20201
ATTN: PRA

and to:
Office of Management and Budget
Paperwork Reduction Project (0910-0291)
Washington, DC 20503

Please do NOT return this form to either of these addresses.

FDA Form 3500A - back

- A string of similar incident types
- Serious medication errors
- Adverse patient care outcomes
- Falls (even without injury)
- Altercations involving physical contact between patients and staff

As many of these conditions suggest, patterns and trends are particularly significant and signal the need for a thorough investigation.

In many ways, a formal investigation mirrors the supervisory informal investigation but on a larger scale. Surveying the scene, talking with those involved, and determining causes are the major elements. If a thorough incident report has been completed, investigators will have less work to do. Much of the information they are seeking deals with the who, what, when, where, and why answered by a well-designed incident report. In addition, they must answer these questions:

- Who had the most control over the conditions surrounding the incident (supervisor, employee, manager)?
- What are the causes of the incident?
- What can be done to prevent recurrence?

As previously mentioned, it is important to remember that incidents have many contributing secondary causes. Examples include:

- Unsafe conditions (chemical hazards, poor housekeeping)
- Unsafe acts (failure to follow procedures or wear proper personal protective equipment)
- Management system deficiencies (inadequate training or staffing levels, lack of procedures)
- Personal factors (tension, fatigue, distraction)

These causes can influence each other. For example, an employee may be tired (personal factor) because the facility is understaffed (management system deficiency) or an employee may not use a safety guard on a power tool (unsafe act) because it malfunctions (unsafe condition). Investigators should realize that, more often than not, causes from each of these categories play a role in the incident.

Additionally, it is important to remember that time is an essential element in the investigation. The investigation must take place as soon as possible after the incident so that facts are fresh in the minds of those involved.

Once the investigation has been completed, a report should be written describing both its methods and results. Again, blame should be avoided; an objective discussion of the cause of the incident will prove much more productive. Most important, the report should include corrective measures, ways to carry them out, and timetables for their implementation. The investigation report will serve as the working reference for the prevention methods introduced as a result of the investigation.

Developing Effective Interviewing Skills

One of the most effective investigative techniques is that of interviewing. The scene of the incident will provide clues as to what occurred and to the conditions that may have contributed to the incident. The greatest source of information is the employee, patient, or other individual involved in the incident. The way to obtain the essential information from this person is through a personal interview.

Interviewing may seem deceptively simple—a few casual questions are asked and straight-forward answers received. Like most human interactions, however, interviewing is more complex than it would appear. Interpersonal factors, fear of reprisal, and numerous other factors can affect the progress and outcome of the interview. In short, interviewing requires specific skills that can be developed through monitoring and practice.

To begin, attention should be paid to the place and time of the interview. The room should not create an atmosphere that is too formal. If possible, a place other than the interviewer's office should be chosen to help the employee understand that the interview is not a disciplinary action. The room should provide privacy, comfort, and freedom from distraction. Calls should be held and visits prevented.

The interviewer should start with some small talk to put the interviewee at ease, and then should say something like "Jeff," (or "Mr. Brown," whichever is appropriate to the relationship) "would you please describe for me in your own words exactly what happened?" The employee or patient should be allowed to tell his or her story without interruption. This avoids influencing the employee's story with questions that lead in a certain direction (for example, "Why was there no label on the container?").

After the interviewee has told his or her story, the interviewer should repeat the story to ensure correct understanding. The interviewer also may want to have the employee or patient pantomime any actions that may be difficult to describe. For example, the interviewer could ask, "Would you mind showing me how you turned to hear what your supervisor was saying?" This may clarify any confusion.

After the story has been told, any gaps or inconsistencies that still remain will be the topic of the interviewer's follow-up questions. Again, the employee's or patient's initial telling of the story should not be interrupted.

One effective interviewing technique is the open-ended question. Open-ended questions require more than a yes or no answer, and often begin with the words *how, what,* and *why.* For example, the interviewer might ask "What did you do next?" or "What did you think then?" rather than "Did you tell your supervisor?" Because open-ended questions allow the interviewee to answer fully, they can provide a wealth of information.

In addition to asking the right kinds of questions, the interviewer should employ effective listening skills. One way to enhance listening is to clear the mind of all extraneous thoughts and concentrate on what the employee or patient is saying. To ensure that he or she has understood the interviewee, the interviewer should repeat or paraphrase what the interviewee has said.

The interviewer also should pay close attention to the emotional content of the speaker's words. People feel that they have been understood when the person they are talking to acknowledges the feelings and frustrations behind their words. Saying things such as "You seem upset," "I know you are worried," or "That must have been frightening" can go a long way toward showing sympathy and understanding. This emotional clarity also will provide clues to the logic and motivations of the person at the time of the incident—information that can be valuable to any investigation.

As the interview draws to a close, the conversation should be directed toward optimism about the future. The interview should always conclude on a positive note. It is important to talk about the work that is being done to prevent such incidents from happening in the future. The interviewer should thank the employee or patient for participating in the interview or "for giving assistance," and should reiterate the concern of management and administration for employee and patient safety and health.

Using Data-Tracking Systems

A comprehensive incident-reporting system that is used routinely by the staff probably will generate extensive amounts of information. However, simply having the information provides no benefits. The success of incident reporting hinges on what is done with the information. Although individual incident reports may have some important uses, additional information is needed for the incident-reporting system to meet its full potential.

Summary data from a number of incidents can uncover conditions difficult to detect even by monitoring every individual incident. For example, incidents that are months apart and in different departments may form part of a year-long pattern that can be detected only with the recordkeeping and computation provided by an organized system of data tracking. Data-tracking systems compile information on numerous variables involved in incidents, such as incident type, time of day, shift, and occupation. In this way, trends and related factors become evident.

These systems do not have to be complex. A log form (figure 12-8) tracks and compares many variables. This kind of form has space to note what corrective actions were taken and

Figure 12-8. Data-Tracking Form

Subject or Department _____

#	Date and Person Reporting	Specific Problem	Contributing Factors	Suggested Solution(s)	Responsible Department	Implementation Date	Results of Action	Next Review Date	Status and Further Action	Next Review Date	Status and Further Action	Date Solved

when, providing the ability to monitor the status of action taken on an incident. A good data-tracking system allows the safety director or person responsible to track and follow up on incidents, and to ensure that action is taken and corrective measures are evaluated for effectiveness. OSHA Form 200 also can be used or adapted for use in this capacity.

Many facilities are turning to computer programs for data analysis, rather than using forms. Often, these systems allow much more detailed analysis and streamline recordkeeping. When purchasing data-tracking programs, the person responsible must ensure that support and training are available from the software company and that all necessary staff members are trained to use the system. This may require patience in overcoming computer phobia. If installing such software is feasible, the facility can reap many benefits. However, smaller facilities with fewer resources can have effective data-tracking systems using regular documentation on well-designed forms.

□ Conclusion

One of the most important elements of incident reporting is the way that incident investigations are conducted. If the causes are not determined and removed, today's near-miss incident could result in tomorrow's serious injury. The purpose of incident investigation is to determine the facts, not to find blame. Effective investigations may include retracing the sequence of events, discovering multiple causes, and interviewing those involved. Incidents may have many causes, and it is important to find all of them in order to prevent accidents from recurring.

□ *Chapter Thirteen*

Training and Development

$\mathbf{I}$n discussions of safety, one word appears more frequently than any other—*training*. Few if any other elements of safety can be considered as crucial to the success of a safety program as ongoing training in safe attitudes and practices. Regulatory and voluntary compliance agency requirements should be enough in themselves to warrant a full-fledged safety training system. Virtually every major law and regulation affecting health care calls for staff education to ensure that employees understand what is required of them and their employer.

Training is the essential element in some standards, for example, the Hazard Communication or Right-to-Know Standard, which mandates that workers have the right to be informed and trained. Regulatory emphasis on training reflects the belief among compliance organizations that facility-sponsored continuing education is the most effective way to ensure that their requirements are met.

Even without emphasis by the Joint Commission on Accreditation of Healthcare Organizations (JCAHO), the Occupational Safety and Health Administration (OSHA), the Environmental Protection Agency (EPA), and numerous other agencies, training would still be intrinsic to the successful operation of a health care facility. As with every learned skill, constant practice and access to instruction represent the only means of ensuring continued capability and expertise in the use of safety techniques. Employees must be helped to understand the need for safety, the concepts underlying program elements, and the techniques of risk avoidance.

Because of its significance, safety training must draw on careful planning and attention to quality. Undoubtedly, the ability to conduct effective, enjoyable training is a skill—and one that can be developed.

This chapter describes a step-by-step approach to developing an effective training program. It also discusses the three levels of training that the health care facility must provide: new employee orientation, current employee training, and management training.

□ Developing a Safety Training Program

Before launching an extensive safety training program, time should be devoted to planning. During the planning phase, efforts should be made to integrate safety education with all other training. Safety then becomes a part of not only every job requirement but also of all job training. The benefit of this integrated approach is that it presents safety as an element of employee job performance, which will be viewed as such by management.

Step-by-Step Approach

Planning successful safety training requires an organized step-by-step process. Some basic steps in planning and evaluating safety training include:

1. *Determine training needs.* Certain topics should be included in all health care safety training: infectious disease hazards, fire prevention, incident reporting, disaster preparedness, hazardous waste disposal, electrical safety, and body mechanics, to name but a few. Many of them already may be part of the facility's training through various departments or in-service education. Tools such as testing, direct observation of performance, and questionnaires can be useful in identifying the facility's specific training needs. In addition, items such as incident reports and statistics on employee injuries can determine the need for education on topics such as body mechanics or correct needle disposal. The facility's needs provide the raw data from which the training program will be developed.

    Deciding what training needs exist also depends on the unique characteristics of the facility staff. Factors such as average age, educational background, area of the country, and previous experience all have a bearing on how much and what type of training is necessary. Training for an older, more experienced staff must focus on performance upgrading that avoids condescension. Safety training for a largely younger staff or for employees in a new facility will start with the basics.

2. *Determine facility capabilities.* Once training needs have been outlined, those responsible for safety programs must determine how the facility can meet these needs. Staff members of health care facilities have widely varying personal and educational backgrounds. This diversity provides a pool of people with different talents and abilities, which often can be used in safety training. Outgoing, involved individuals may be chosen to be instructors. Creative employees may help to write program materials or design audiovisual materials. Technical experts can review content. Many health care facilities find that using these staff resources greatly enhances training quality and employee participation.

    Not every facility can or should undertake all training in-house. There are innumerable outside resources, and not all of them are costly. For example, consultants may be used to design and instruct in-service education. Associations to which the facility belongs may provide materials or assistance. Relatively inexpensive written training programs are available to minimize development time and cost. Whatever the facility's resources, high-quality, cost-effective training is feasible.

3. *Assign training responsibilities.* To ensure an organized program, someone should be designated to coordinate all safety training. The safety training coordinator should possess both interest and experience in training and in safety. Moreover, he or she must be capable of working with other departments. This process encourages greater integration of safety and job training.

    In addition to the appointment of a safety training coordinator, individuals should be chosen for other aspects of training. On the basis of staff resources identified when determining facility capabilities, individuals should be chosen to be course instructors, to help write and develop programs, to plan room arrangements, and to conduct other necessary tasks in planning and implementing safety training.

4. *Design the program.* Once the preceding steps have been accomplished, it will be relatively easy to design and prioritize training—that is, how the learning needs will be met (audiovisual aids, study guides, team activities, lectures), who the instructor or presenter will be, and how to determine when the needs have been met (practice with coaching, testing, observing, feedback).

5. *Carry out the training.* Attention to detail is important. Seating should be arranged to facilitate interaction. The room—chairs, air temperature, noise level—should be comfortable and conducive to learning. Breaks should be given and, where the session is long or includes a meal hour, refreshments should be provided.

6. *Evaluate the training and revise it accordingly.* The success and effectiveness of the educational session should be determined so that future training can improve, if necessary. Many techniques can be used to determine what employees learned and what they liked and disliked about the program. Using techniques such as giving tests before

and after the program, providing evaluation forms (figure 13-1), and monitoring employee practices after the training can be helpful. Ongoing reinforcement stimulates commitment and pride among employees. For example, 10-minute briefings, minitraining programs, and updates such as newsletters can be very effective as ongoing reinforcement.

7. *Plan for updated training programs when necessary.* Because of the high likelihood for changes in regulations and safety needs, evaluations should be conducted at regular intervals to determine additional training needs. Changes in procedures, new equipment, and regulations may require employees to undergo further training to update their knowledge.

Figure 13-1. Sample Training Evaluation Form

1. Topic and date of in-service: _____

2. Overall rating of in-service (1–10: 1 = worst; 10 = best): _____

3. Rating of instructor (1–10) in the following categories:

    Preparation _____

    Content of presentation _____

    Speaking ability _____

    Responsiveness to audience _____

    Other (please list) _____

4. What did you like *most* about the in-service? _____
    _____

5. What did you like *least* about the in-service? _____
    _____

6. What information did you find most valuable? _____
    _____

7. Do you have any suggestions for changes or improvements, or any other comments? Please list (use back of form if necessary). _____
    _____
    _____
    _____

8. Please list your department. _____

9. What departmental issues or other topics would you like to see covered in future in-services? _____
    _____
    _____

Thank you for taking the time to fill out this form. If any of your concerns cannot be addressed using this form, feel free to discuss them with the instructors and (person responsible for the training). We value your opinion, and your comments and suggestions will be used in designing future training and educational programs.

Sincerely,

(Signature of person responsible for the training)

Basic Training Program Components

Although *every* facility has its own unique needs and priorities, some basic components should be included in any safety training program. These are:

- Explanation of the facility's safety program (components, staff, resources, and so on)
- Explanations of pertinent regulations and how to comply
- Hazardous and infectious materials handling
- Accident prevention techniques, such as back injury prevention and electrical safety precautions
- Fire protection methods
- Patient safety
- Emergency preparedness
- Use of personal protective equipment (PPE)
- Accident reporting
- Information on resources available to employees, such as the facility's safety committee and material safety data sheets
- Infection control precautions, including AIDS/hepatitis B virus (HBV) protection

These represent minimum safety training topics. Others chosen will depend on individual facility needs, problems experienced, and state and local regulations.

Regulatory Requirements

Another important factor in safety training is providing training for regulatory requirements. Each level of training should include appropriate safety and regulatory information for that particular level.

Both OSHA and the EPA have specific employee safety training requirements, as do other regulatory agencies. Some OSHA regulations mandate training frequency as well, especially for employees who may be exposed to certain toxic chemicals. Under OSHA regulations, employers must provide employees with training and education programs in addition to pertinent job information. This information includes:

- Proper working conditions and precautions
- Possible exposure to hazards on the job
- Symptoms of toxic exposure to substances in the workplace
- Emergency treatment procedures

OSHA also gives specific suggestions for management and supervisory training. This includes an explanation of supervisory responsibility for:

- Analyzing the work supervised to identify unrecognized potential hazards
- Maintaining PPE in the respective work areas
- Providing and reinforcing employee training on the nature of potential occupational hazards in the facility and on necessary protective measures to control exposures

Compliance with these and other regulations is of utmost importance in a safety training program. Planning of the safety program should include thorough review to ensure that all regulatory requirements are met.

Training Methods and Strategies

At *every* level of training, knowingly or not, instructors use some type of training method or strategy. In many cases, the strategy is as simple as a classroom lecture. Although this teaching method can be effective, trainers should be aware of the wide array of other techniques available for the enhancement of learning. Also, lecture has several disadvantages when used alone and may be inappropriate for many learning situations and audience needs.

A number of commonly used training techniques can boost the success of in-service and other training. These techniques include:

- *Discussion:* The instructor facilitates discussion with and among the students. Discussion is useful for encouraging participatory learning and for gathering ideas and solving problems creatively.
- *Demonstration/skills training:* The instructor acts out steps to be learned, repeating the procedure with learner input. An example of this strategy is the step-by-step technique outlined in the employee training section (discussed later in this chapter). This is quite effective in teaching a skill.
- *Role-playing:* During role-playing, the instructor assigns participants parts to play. Often the circumstances for role-playing are scenarios that test what already has been learned. For example, in an in-service session on interviewing skills for accident investigators, one student might play an injured patient and another the safety director. This technique reinforces learning and allows students to understand the real-life roles of other personnel in the facility.
- *Brainstorming:* Like discussion, brainstorming relies on verbal interaction. All group members are allowed to suggest any ideas that come to mind, however odd or irrelevant. Brainstorming often generates many valuable options during problem solving.
- *Case study:* This approach consists of reading (or viewing on a videotape) a realistic situation and responding to it. For example, a disaster involving a tornado, several hundred community casualties, and loss of electricity could be described. Employees from different departments would then explain step-by-step what they would do in this case. This method has wide applicability in teaching incident reporting, emergency preparedness, hazardous chemicals procedures, and so on.
- *Self-study:* This method uses programmed lessons and exercises that the student studies individually. The instructor then follows up with group discussion and perhaps reinforcement testing. Self-study allows all students to progress at their own pace. However, students must be motivated to complete lessons on their own.

These techniques represent a few of the major training strategies. Others include audiovisual materials (audiotapes, videotapes, overhead transparencies, charts), learning games, questioning, class exercises, listening tests, and handouts. The number and type of techniques possible are limited only by the trainer's imagination.

Additional creative training approaches reinforce learning and communication. The skills employees learn can be designed to improve people-interaction ability. Safety training sessions can include:

- Handling difficult situations
- Improving listening skills
- Learning how to go the extra step to solve a problem
- Understanding how our own behavior affects the way others see us
- Increasing communication among departments

Creative approaches include:

- *Music:* By the proper use of music in training, learning takes on a new dimension. Music affects emotions and motivation.
- *Reflections:* Self-image is important. Training helps employees understand that what they think about themselves is as important as what others think about them.

- *Listening:* Learning how to solve employee or patient problems requires listening to what they are saying and why it's important to them. Many times what someone is saying is not exactly what they mean. By teaching good listening skills, employees will be able to empathize with others.
- *Choosing emotions:* During training employees can be placed in situations that teach them about emotional reactions. They learn to solve problems effectively without becoming emotionally involved. Training can show them how to find and implement the most effective solutions.
- *Surprises:* Unexpected situations can occur in training that require employees to practice the skills they are learning. These situations stimulate surprises that can occur when they are working. Someone who is prepared handles situations better than someone who has never seen the situation before.
- *All-the-time skills:* Employees appreciate acquiring skills that they can use at home as well as at work. Behavior cannot be turned on and off depending on the surrounding environment—work or home. Learning how to utilize service skills in everyday life helps make the skills an integral part of employees' personalities.

There are certain other factors that will influence training methods used. Principal among these is *cost.* For example, cost differs for various techniques. Advanced audiovisual materials such as interactive video will cost more than informal group discussion. Similarly, having a year of in-service sessions designed and instructed by a consultant may involve more expense than purchasing one interactive video.

Drawing on staff ingenuity, some training needs can be creatively filled in-house. For example, some facilities have written and directed their own training videos, often with great success. Although not always of the highest quality, these videos can help employees understand the materials more clearly because they visualize the procedure.

Another factor that influences training methods is *audience.* Trainers always must consider audience characteristics (background, age, education) and gear training to suit them. For instance, self-study may not be effective when employees are not motivated to work on their own, and role-playing and other games have limited applicability with more mature employees, who may consider them childish. (See figure 13-2 for guidelines on selecting teaching methods.)

Training techniques chosen should not be too conservative but, at the same time, they need to target the audience. The appropriate use of inventive training strategies not only increases

Figure 13-2. Guidelines for Selecting a Teaching Method

- Determine facility resources—staff, funds, time.
- Decide which options will fit within budget restrictions.
- Determine the appropriate method for the audience.
- Match the technique to training needs. For example, skills training requires hands-on learning, but explaining a new regulation may only require lecture and discussion.
- Apply new teaching methods gradually and with explanation, especially for groups accustomed to lecture only.
- Choose only those techniques with which you, the trainer, are comfortable. If you feel awkward or inadequate using a specific method, avoid it until your experience level allows you to feel more comfortable with the strategy. When you are having difficulty, the students will perceive it and may take your instruction less seriously.
- Use only the audiovisual materials that relate to the topic at hand. Avoid the use of films or videotapes as entertainment only. Provide ample time before and after any audiovisual aid to discuss it, and help the audience integrate the material. The audiovisual aid should seldom, if ever, be the focus of the entire training period.
- Preview all audiovisual materials and read all written training materials before discussing them with the class.
- Learn from mistakes and bad choices of training methods, using student evaluation forms.

the volume of what is learned and later practiced, but also makes training a much more enjoyable experience for everyone involved—even new trainers.

☐ Implementing Different Levels of Training

In planning and implementing practical safety training, it should be recognized that different positions in the health care hierarchy require distinct approaches. The three levels of training that should be treated separately are new employee orientation, current employee training, and management training.

New Employee Orientation

Emphasis on safety begins during the employee's first contacts with the organization—hiring and orientation. All new employees want to feel accepted. Trainers can respond to that desire during the orientation process.

By gathering all new employees together, the trainer helps each employee feel less conspicuous. Supervisors and other trainers should welcome new employees in a friendly and personal way. They should emphasize that safety is a major part of the facility's philosophy and everyday operation. Safe actions can be presented as a way to "fit in," and participation in safety programs can be presented as one method of becoming an established member of the facility's team.

Orientation must cover many topics in order to serve its purpose of welcoming employees and helping them come up to the facility's standards. There are a multitude of questions in the minds of new employees, especially about terms of employment. Sick days, vacation, benefits, and other vital information should be communicated early in the orientation. With these questions answered, new employees will feel more at ease and be open to absorbing other information.

Orientation safety training should include an introduction to each of the minimum elements of safety. In this way, groundwork is laid not only for safe practices early in the employee's term of service but also for later safety training. The introduction must remain general in order to allow for time to cover each topic. Informal training on the job, as well as later in-service training, will fill in details.

Finally, orientation represents the ideal time for upper-level management to demonstrate its support for the safety program. Top management can do this by attending the safety orientation part of the program. Management should reiterate the welcome that other personnel have extended and emphasize the significance of safe job performance. At the same time, upper-level management can briefly outline management's efforts, such as the safety program and incentives, to protect the health and safety of the facility's most valuable resource—its employees.

Current Employee Training

Whereas new employee orientation is designed to introduce and underscore the significance of the overall safety program, current employee in-service or educational courses will explain how these measures are actually carried out. Emphasis in ongoing employee training is on skills—developing and reinforcing the procedures that form the foundation of the safety program.

It is very important that training be a rewarding experience for the employees involved. Trainers should link the training directly to the employees' jobs and daily routine. This gives employees a connection with the training and helps them better assimilate the information. More important, training should not be a burden on employees. Adjustments should be made in work schedules to accommodate the needed time for training. If employees feel the training is a waste of time, they will not be able to concentrate fully on the course and may even resent the time spent in training.

Skills training differs from *routine information dissemination* in that the teaching of skills is less didactic and passive. Skills training requires interaction and two-way communication, whereas routine information dissemination often is lecture based. The trainer must first explain the reasons for methods and their benefits. In helping an employee learn a skill, his or her participation is crucial. Following is an effective step-by-step method for employee training:

1. *Discuss the policy underlying the procedure.* For example, the instructor could explain that accident prevention is a prominent part of the safety program. Because incident reporting can be used to prevent future accidents, incident-reporting methods must be taught to all employees. At the outset, it is important to establish the reason for learning a skill and how that skill will help employees.
2. *Give employees the information they will need to undertake the procedure.* In the case of incident reporting, for instance, the instructor would distribute and explain the report form used by the facility and discuss reportable occurrences.
3. *Explain the steps of the process.* Breaking the skill into manageable steps assists in comprehension.
4. *Demonstrate the skill.* For incident reporting, the instructor could discuss an incident scenario and show (on an overhead transparency) how it would be reported.
5. *Repeat the demonstration, but with feedback.* For example, the instructor could ask employees: "What would I do next?" "What should I write here?"
6. *Supervise practice.* With the example of incident reporting, employees could be divided into groups and given a case study or scenario to react to as if it had happened to them. The instructor would facilitate interaction but remain uninvolved at this stage.
7. *Discuss and review.* The instructor should discuss the case and reports that have been completed, encouraging employees to ask questions. Comments and suggestions should be encouraged. With employee input, the reasoning behind actions and the steps involved could be reviewed. Instructors should hand out evaluation forms and revise the training program as necessary. In addition to certificates, small incentive tokens can be given at the end of each training course. Items such as coffee mugs or paperweights bearing slogans such as Safety Is Our Goal or I Am a Safety Achiever provide recognition and are a daily reminder of the importance of safety.
8. *Reward completion of training.* Personal recognition of achievement perhaps is the most important part of any training program. People like to be rewarded for a job well done. For this reason, employees who have successfully completed a training course should be given some form of recognition. Issuing certificates of completion to employees is a way to thank them for their time and effort, and also provides visual commendation. If possible, certificates should be awarded during a short ceremony in the presence of coworkers. This gives the employee a feeling of pride and accomplishment, while providing motivation for other employees who have not yet completed the training.
9. *Document all training in personnel files.* Documentation is important for proof of compliance and staff competence.

This step-by-step process requires trainers to explain what will be taught, to teach the materials, and to review what was learned. It emphasizes learning a skill and understanding the philosophy behind it. Finally, it allows for interaction and employee input—elements that have been shown to increase the probability that new skills will be used in everyday job performance.

Management Training

Training those who will manage employees requires a carefully designed approach. Management training will center less on developing skills than on helping others to cultivate them. Because of their crucial role in ensuring that safety practices are followed, managers must be taught how to train.

This "train-the-trainer" approach consists of a number of elements. As with employee training, conceptual information comes first. Management must be fully versed in all components of regulatory policies and procedures. It is important that managers fully understand these concepts before they explain them to their employees. Managers also should be taught how to explain regulations to their employees and how to detect unsafe acts. Other important concepts to cover include the origin of and reasons for the safety program, the need for each element, and management's role in the program's effective operation.

Although it is important to demonstrate the program's benefits to the manager, it is equally important to emphasize its benefits to the entire facility. Safety should be tied to the facility's mission and to its formal performance evaluation system.

Supervisors and managers need not be instructors in the formal safety program to be considered trainers. Their routine management responsibilities require constant training of employees. Each time they demonstrate a technique or praise or criticize an employee, they are involved in training. As a result, managers wield the most control over what employees learn to do. Managers should realize during training that this influence can be used to teach and encourage safe procedures, which will protect the employee, the department, and the facility as a whole.

Although managers may be pleased by the importance of their role, they also may feel inadequate as trainers—particularly if their responsibilities will include formal classroom instruction. To alleviate this feeling of inadequacy, managers should receive instruction in training methods, including public speaking, communication, and techniques to enliven the training process. This brief instruction will empower managers to be more effective trainers and will thus enhance the quality of training the employees receive. (See figure 13-3 for helpful hints for beginning trainers/teachers.)

It may not be possible to accomplish all of the above through in-service training or other in-house instruction. Therefore, professional development of managers should be encouraged

Figure 13-3. Helpful Hints for Beginning Trainers

- *Flexibility* is important in the classroom. Students may become excited about an issue or portion of content. Encourage discussion even though the issues may not be part of the lesson plan or do not cover specific objectives. Individuals may be stimulated to research further information and become involved in further sessions.

- *Variety* may be introduced by providing for a number of different activities. Learners remain alert and become responsive when there is an exciting and stimulating environment in the classroom.

- Provide for some *personal time* for each learner.

- Offer *approval*, a nod, a smile for good work done.

- Student *self-evaluations* are often helpful. A positive approach should be used and an outline given. Items such as: "What have you learned and in what areas have you achieved success?" and "In what areas do you need more assistance?" are items which need to be explored.

- Provide for *eye contact*. Look at each student many times. Faces which demonstrate a frown, preoccupied look, or panic in taking notes offer a strong clue that some students are lost in the learning process.

- Ask for student *assistance* and *analysis* as to what went on in the classroom. Did you break the monotony or specific train of thought by using an audiovisual aid? How did the group respond?

- *Participative learning* gets adults actively involved in the teaching–learning process.

- *Answer* all questions asked. Adults must not hesitate to ask questions by thinking that perhaps the questions are not good ones or that their peers have the answers.

- *Preview* all *materials* before presenting them to the class. If you are unclear on any points, research them to gain better understanding. This will better prepare you for possible questions from the students.

- *Encourage questions* from students through your reactions. Comments like "That's a good question" can put students at ease about asking for further clarification on a topic.

- Periodically *ask* the *students* if they have any questions, particularly if none have been presented. This allows students the opportunity to clarify points they might not have understood during the presentation.

- Allow for *breaks* if the course is going to last for an extended period.

- Make training *enjoyable*. Students will look forward to learning, and will retain the new information longer.

Adapted from Dyche, J. *Educational Program Development for Employees in Health Care Agencies.* Los Angeles: Tri-Oak Educational Division, 1982, p. 51.

through outside conferences, seminars, and so on. Many associations and professional groups offer courses for continuing education credit. The investment will pay off when supervisors and managers can conduct effective and enjoyable training, minimizing the need for outside speakers and reducing the overall cost of high-quality training. Finally, as with all other instruction, management training should be evaluated and documented.

☐ Working Successfully with Other Departments

Just as integrating safety into other training is essential to establishing the importance of safety, so is cooperation among departments. The safety department, or other responsible department, cannot act alone in developing and implementing safety training. Often, the resulting program will be viewed by employees as something unnecessary and unrelated to them. Without departmental interaction, individual department safety training needs often are not met.

Consequently, safety trainers should consult with all departments in designing training. For example, the safety director can meet with the nursing administrator to ask for input. What are nursing's safety training priorities? What do nursing personnel see as vital to the protection of the facility? The safety director can invite the nursing administrator and department managers to participate in program development, such as teaching the medication error session, developing the AIDS/HBV protection lesson, and so on. Often an invitation to assist in training will generate commitment among other departments to the safety training program.

Those with safety training responsibilities also should work with department managers and employees to design targeted training sessions. These in-service sessions are geared toward solving specific problems that have been identified in a department, such as a rash of patient falls or hazardous chemical spills. When managers and employees in departments see that safety training can benefit them by solving their individual problems, their commitment and participation in facilitywide training will grow. It is then that safety training can become an effective and adaptive force for employee and facility protection alike.

☐ Conclusion

Safety training is one of the most crucial elements to the success of a safety program. Employees must be trained in safe attitudes and practices not only to minimize incidents, but also to comply with state and federal regulatory requirements. Safety training is necessary for all levels of employees, from new employees to management. Careful planning and consistent evaluation help ensure that safety training is thorough and up-to-date. Through proper evaluation, training efficiency can be measured and adjustments made where necessary. Good training produces workers who are skilled and productive—as well as safe.

Special Considerations in Mental Health Settings

Due to growing public awareness and concern, mental health institutions and psychiatric units in general health care facilities are targets of tightening regulatory controls in the area of safety. In order to ensure a safe, workable mental health setting, patient violence, suicide, and elopement must be dealt with and safety policies and procedures implemented.

This chapter discusses the special considerations that mental health facilities must take into account in developing safety policies and procedures. It also describes inspection guidelines that facilities must follow to ensure compliance with various regulatory standards.

☐ Safety Policies and Procedures

Preventing accidents is a high-priority need in mental health facilities. Individuals responsible for facility or departmental safety need to develop and implement safety policies and procedures to keep accidents to a minimum. Once implemented, policies and procedures should be reviewed on a regular basis and revised as needed.

Among the unique risks that health care facilities must consider in developing their safety policies and procedures are patient violence, suicide, and elopement. The following subsections examine these risks.

Violence and Suicide

Because they sometimes are disoriented and fearful, mentally ill patients can respond to otherwise harmless or mildly irritating incidents as if they were threats. In some cases, anger or thoughts of self-destruction may develop as a result of being hospitalized, causing patients to behave violently or to attempt suicide. Thus, to be in a position to determine potentially dangerous patient behavior, the facility must develop a policy describing assessment and monitoring criteria. The policy should include:

- Consideration of the facility's capabilities to adequately protect patients, employees, and visitors from dangerous patients. For example, in mental health units of general health care facilities in which structural security and trained staff members may not be sufficient to protect personnel, patients, and the community, procedures should be outlined for transferring patients to an appropriate facility, when necessary.
- Criteria for determining potential danger of patient upon admission and regularly thereafter. Indicators of potential danger include:
  —Previous assaults or destructive behavior
  —Threats of violence or suicide

———Chaotic family life
———Alcohol/drug use
———Posttraumatic stress disorder (PTSD)
———History of abuse or abusiveness
———Hostile feelings
———Severe environmental stressors
- Provision for closely monitoring suicidal or destructive patients.
- A procedure for transferring patients to a designated control or holding room, and a description of how this room should be maintained. For example, the room should not contain items that can be used as weapons (for example, plastic trash can liners and glass mirrors, or shower heads and rods capable of supporting body weight).
- Directions for checking patients every 15 minutes and for documenting the checks.
- Provision for maintaining patients committed to a control or holding room. For example, all straps and ties should be removed from patient clothing; patient belongings should be checked for items that could be used for self-injury; patients should be given finger foods.
- A procedure requiring that all suicides and attempted suicides be documented in incident reports and investigated.
- A procedure defining security measures to be enacted when dealing with outpatients.
- A procedure ensuring that patients cannot obtain contraband. Patient body cavity searches are not routine, but may need to be considered by medical staff in extraordinary circumstances.
- Provision for checking visitors for weapons, drugs, and so on.

Elopement

Patient escape to the outside is always a concern in mental health settings. In addition to the harm that an escaped patient could do to himself or herself and others, elopement has the potential of generating adverse publicity and protest from the community. Additionally, the facility can be held accountable for the actions of an escaped patient, particularly a criminal patient or one who was committed involuntarily. Consequently, the facility must enact stringent security measures to conform to local laws. The facility or the unit safety staff should establish a healthy, cooperative relationship with the community security force. Security personnel can act as a valuable resource, particularly when made aware of the special needs of psychiatric patients. The facility should be designed to be secure, and inspections should be conducted regularly to ensure its continuing security.

In some circumstances, patients may have periodic leave rights. Thus, staff should be familiar with the laws and regulations regarding involuntary and voluntary detention.

At the same time, every attempt should be made to provide a pleasant and unrestricted atmosphere for patients. They should be provided with ample recreation consistent with treatment goals, and visits with family and friends should be encouraged.

☐ Safety Inspection Guidelines

Local and state agencies require mental health units and facilities to comply with stringent safety regulations and inspections in order to ensure that patients are provided with exceptional care and a safe environment. Facilities should conduct regular inspections to ensure their compliance with these requirements. (Standards may differ in each location, and individual facilities should check with regional agencies when planning an inspection.) Guidelines for the inspection should include safety concerns for the general psychiatric unit or facility, patient rooms, and control or holding rooms.

General Psychiatric Unit or Facility

General psychiatric units and facilities should be inspected to ensure that they meet a number of safety precautions. These include the following:

- Exit doors should be equipped with alarms.
- Fire pull boxes should be tamper-resistant or equipped with alarms.
- Fire extinguishers should be used in place of fire hoses, if possible, and should be in recessed, tamper-resistant boxes.
- Security doors should be equipped with alarms.
- Chute doors should be designed to prevent accidental entrance or injury.
- Windows should be made of safety glass that can withstand substantial force.
- Screws (including those used on electrical faceplates) should be tamper-resistant and require a special tool for removal.
- Base coving should be avoided because it can be used as a hiding place for contraband.
- Newly installed furniture, carpeting, and fabrics should be Class 1 or Class A fire-resistant.
- Cleaning supplies should be secured at all times.
- Housekeeping carts should not be left unattended.
- Sharps containers should be kept locked in nursing stations.

Patient Rooms

Because of the constant potential for sudden violence and suicide attempts by patients, special care should be taken in designing and maintaining patient rooms. Some essential considerations include:

- Mirrors should not contain glass. Instead, they should be made of acrylic plastic or stainless steel and should be firmly mounted to a structural wall.
- Light fixtures should be recessed and secured with tamperproof screws.
- Shower rods, shower heads, towel racks, clothing racks, and other items strong enough to support body weight should be of the breakaway type or made of soft, bendable material such as polyvinyl chloride (PVC) piping. Shower heads should be recessed so that cords and pipes are not available for destructive use. The facility must take into consideration that items unable to support average adult body weight may be able to support the weight of children, adolescents, or small-framed adults. Therefore, if the facility treats patients who fit these categories, additional precautions should be taken.
- Loose structural elements such as shelving or ledges should be removed or tightly secured.
- Flowerpots and vases should be made of plastic. (Consideration should be given to not allowing the use of *any* flower pots and vases in a patient room. These objects can be thrown or broken apart and used as a sharp object.)
- Three-pronged ground-fault circuit interrupter (GFCI) safety outlets should be used.
- Plastic bags, including trash can liners, should not be placed or allowed in patient rooms.
- Ropes and strings (including drawstrings for drapery) should be removed.
- Rooms should be checked regularly and thoroughly for dangerous items that patients may have hidden, including sharp objects, rope, and plastic bags.
- Windows should be secured and made of safety glass.
- Rooms should not have drop or tile ceilings. Ceilings should be of solid construction.
- Furniture should be secured to walls and/or floors, or be of sufficient weight that it cannot be easily moved or picked up by the patient.

Control or Holding Rooms

Most psychiatric units and facilities have safe rooms where aggressive or suicidal patients may be held. Even the most seemingly innocuous items in these rooms can pose a serious safety hazard to patients desperate enough to hurt themselves or others. Consequently, these rooms should be designed to protect patients and others in the facility and community.

In addition to the safety measures normally required for patient rooms, the design of control or holding rooms must take into account special precautions. For example:

- Beds should be equipped with a molded foam rubber mattress and a nonmetal box spring and have no other framing.
- Any windows should be heavily protected.
- The room shape should include as few protruding corners as possible.
- The door should be made of bonded wood core or other approved material, and should contain a wire glass window for monitoring the patient.
- If a closed-circuit television camera with a remote monitor is installed to assist in monitoring, it should be recessed or positioned out of patient reach. If it cannot be recessed, a secured steel casing should surround the camera. An intercom should be installed to enable communication between staff members and patient.
- Standard ½- or ⅝-inch-thick walls and ceilings may have to be reinforced as the standard thicknesses may allow a patient to break through.
- Bathrooms inside the rooms should not be lockable from the inside unless there is an emergency override on the outside and the door swings both ways.
- Air vents should be incapable of supporting body weight.
- Rooms should not have drop or tile ceilings. Ceilings should be of solid construction.

☐ Conclusion

Like other health care facilities, mental health units and institutions assume responsibility for maintaining a safe and secure environment for patients, families, and employees. Therefore, all the safety elements described previously in this text should be incorporated in mental health settings in health care facilities and mental health facilities' overall safety programs—emergency preparedness, fire safety, departmental safety, and patient safety, to name a few. In addition, mental health facilities must take some special precautions to ensure the safety of their patient populations. Three unique risks that facilities must consider in developing safety policies and procedures are violence, suicide, and elopement. By implementing a comprehensive safety and risk reduction program, the facility will ensure its ability to meet accelerating demands while providing a safe, risk-free environment.

Safety Motivational Programs

S afety motivational programs are an integral part of the health care facility's comprehensive safety program. Properly designed, they augment the fundamental safety programs by creating safety awareness and positive reinforcement of good safety performance. Moreover, they encourage employees to make a long-term commitment to safety and remind them of the value of their contributions and of opportunities for continued recognition.

This chapter discusses the two basic types of safety motivational programs—promotional programs and incentive programs. It also describes safety recognition organizations and off-the-job safety programs.

☐ Promotional Programs

Promotion is to safety what advertising is to the sale of a product. By making customers aware of a product's value, advertising motivates them to buy it. Safety promotion makes employees aware of the value of safety to themselves and their families, and motivates them to create and maintain an injury-free environment.

Promotional programs build employee excitement and create awareness of the facility's programs, goals, and accomplishments. A program promoting safety requires an aggressive campaign delivered in a variety of ways to make safety visible to employees at all times. Visibility can be accomplished in a number of ways, including:

- High-visibility celebrations of milestones using awards, parties, and congratulatory messages
- Themes and logos that provide a unique identity and tie all the safety programs together
- Safety contests and awards programs
- Notices announcing employee accomplishments on bulletin boards and in other visible ways
- Safety information telephone hotlines
- Electronic message boards
- Safety newsletters
- Motivational and informational posters
- Annual safety kickoff meetings to review past performance and goals for the coming year

In addition to the promotional techniques listed above, products such as key chains, coffee mugs, calendars, and T-shirts can serve as rewards, as well as daily reminders of the importance of safety (because recipients usually keep them for a long time). A survey conducted of travelers at Chicago's O'Hare International Airport by Promotional Products Association

International showed that 67 percent of employees used promotional items for more than one year and 21 percent kept them for six months to one year.

☐ Incentive Programs

Incentive programs build employee motivation by recognizing and rewarding outstanding safety performance and the achievement of specific goals. They have the greatest impact when they focus on specific safety performance objectives. Although programs that reward employees for minimal contribution may meet the objective of promoting safety awareness, they usually contribute little to improve long-term safety performance or to correct specific safety problems.

Successful incentive programs may be characterized in one or more ways. For example:

- They are goal oriented and focus on correcting and improving safety performance. Examples of program goals include:
  —To reduce the frequency of specific injuries, such as needle sticks or slips and falls, by 50 percent
  —To state 100 percent adherence to safety rules and procedures during inspectional walk-throughs
  —To increase employee knowledge of safety rules to a score of at least 80 percent on knowledge-retention tests
- They recognize individuals or groups for work outside their normal assignment—for example, employee contribution to a specific safety project or participation on a safety committee.
- They offer rewards that are relatively difficult to obtain but are achievable by those employees willing to become involved.
- They involve employees as much as possible in safety program development and implementation.
- They instill in employees feelings of pride and job satisfaction through management and peer group recognition.
- They are highly publicized before, during, and after the life of the program.
- They are easy to understand and implement.

Criteria for Selecting an Incentive Program

Safety incentive programs should be managed in the same manner as other programs, with an eye toward cost reduction, quality improvement, and productivity. Program goals, priorities, timing, cost, resources, and assignment of responsibility are key items to consider during program development.

Because there usually is a limit on available resources and funds, it is important to choose programs that focus on significant safety needs. One approach that can be used to choose a program is to identify the most serious safety problems and rank them based on their impact on safety performance. Normally, the safety committee maintains a list of safety priorities and is responsible for evaluating and selecting safety programs. However, departments also can use this process to set up their own incentive programs.

Once a program has been chosen, responsibility for its development usually is given to a committee composed of employees familiar with the problem that the program is supposed to address. In developing the program, the committee should first consider the following questions:

- What are the goals of the program?
- How will accomplishment of these goals be measured?
- Who needs to participate in the program to accomplish its goals?
- What type of incentive award should be given?

- How long will the program last?
- What must program participants accomplish to earn the award?
- How much will awards cost and how will they be funded?

To facilitate this process, the committee should survey employees to obtain their ideas and suggestions.

Examples of Prepared Programs

Incentive programs often are developed in-house and tailored to tie in with specific goals and objectives. However, considerable time can be saved by using other facilities' programs that have proven successful in achieving specific goals. Prepared programs can also be obtained from safety promotion companies.

A number of incentive programs have been used successfully to improve safety performance. Following are descriptions of four of them:

Employee-of-the-Month Award

The goal of this program is to motivate employees by recognizing individual safety accomplishments. Employee input into the program is used to create interest and excitement. Each month, employees nominate coworkers who they feel have made a valuable contribution to safety. A safety award committee then narrows down the list of nominees to a group of finalists from which one is selected as safety employee of the month. A plaque or poster with the employee's picture is then placed in an area designated for safety recognition.

Monthly Recognition Program

The goal of this program is to reduce safety rule violations by recognizing groups that have recorded no safety violations for the month. A safety inspection team inspects the areas regularly and records safety violations. The groups having no violations recorded for the month have their names engraved on a plaque that is then put on public display. This program also inspires a feeling of teamwork and, in some cases, fosters competition among groups with similar duties.

Safety Pin Awards

Many companies award safety pins to employees who complete a set number of years without injury. Annual injury-free awards usually are presented to individuals by department heads. Five-year injury-free awards are given with greater fanfare and publicity. Facilities that are members of the National Safety Council (NSC) can participate in its program called The Safe Worker Award Program. In addition to safety pins, this program offers a variety of other recognition items that can be used to honor milestones in an employee's safety career.

Safety Suggestion Program

The goal of a safety suggestion program is to reduce unsafe conditions by encouraging employees to identify and report them. This program promotes the awareness that safety is the personal responsibility of every employee.

The employee is recognized by a letter of appreciation that also describes the status of the corrective action to be taken. At the end of a six- to twelve-month period, a safety awards committee recognizes employees whose suggestions have made a significant contribution to the safety program. A variation is to conduct quarterly drawings in which each employee who submits a safety suggestion is eligible for a safety prize.

155

☐ Safety Recognition Organizations

Several organizations have established programs to reward individuals for working in a safe manner. These programs are available at modest cost and provide excellent opportunities to publicize safety performance. (See appendix A for a list of some of the organizations that offer such programs.) The following subsections describe three such programs.

The Golden Shoe Club

The Golden Shoe Club Award is made to employees who have prevented injuries to their feet by wearing safety shoes. Maintenance departments frequently use this program to increase employee awareness of the need to wear safety shoes at all times. Any employee who reports an authentic case where foot injury has been avoided by wearing safety shoes is eligible for the award. Information on this program can be obtained from the Hy-Test Division of the International Shoe Company.

The Wise Owl Program

The Wise Owl Program was founded in 1948 to recognize individuals in all types of businesses who avoid eye injury by wearing eye protection. Any organization or company can obtain a charter for a minimal initiation fee. Employees can qualify for a recognition award in one of two ways: They must either conscientiously and routinely wear eye protection or have saved their eyesight by wearing protective equipment during an accident. Information on this program can be obtained from the National Society to Prevent Blindness.

The Golden Belt Club

This award recognizes employees or their families for wearing safety belts at the time of a motor vehicle accident. Information on this program can be obtained from the NSC.

☐ Off-the-Job Safety Programs

Most employee injuries do not occur at work. Table 15-1 shows that workers are almost four times as likely to be killed off the job than on the job. The data also show that workers experience approximately 45 percent more injuries off the job than on the job. One of the reasons for higher off-the-job injury rates is that employee exposure time to injury is almost double the exposure time on the job. Injuries can occur when employees are at home, on the road, or playing sports. This fact makes it extremely important that every facility consider implementing an effective off-the-job safety program. Off-the-job programs pay off in two ways: First and most important, they can reduce injury and suffering to employees and their families; and second, they can significantly reduce cost to the facility in lost time and disability pay.

On- and off-the-job injuries are both caused by the same fundamental problem—unsafe acts and conditions. Unfortunately, by itself, on-the-job safety training does not always translate

Table 15-1. Accidental Deaths and Disabling Injuries

Class of Accident	Severity	One Every	Total 1992
Work	Deaths	62 minutes	8,500
	Injuries	10 seconds	3,300,000
Workers off the job	Deaths	17 minutes	31,400
	Injuries	07 seconds	4,800,000

Source: *Accident Facts 1993 Edition.* Chicago: National Safety Council, 1993.

into improved off-the-job safety performance. However, off-the-job safety awareness programs can be used to extend employee thinking beyond the workplace and into the home.

The NSC conducted a survey of four major corporations to determine the top 10 categories of disabling off-the-job injuries. (See table 15-2.) These data can be used to develop specific topics for safety emphasis programs. Another approach may be to determine the facility's major off-the-job injuries over the past few years and tailor programs based on this information. Topics differ according to time of year and whether emphasis is needed for traffic, home, or other types of injury. (See table 15-3.)

Once a list of topics has been developed, programs can be carried out in much the same manner as on-the-job promotional programs. However, a key difference in the two programs is the need to involve employees' families. Therefore, information about promotional programs (in the form of letters, safety magazines, and so on) should be sent to employees' homes. At work, off-the-job safety programs should be integrated into on-the-job meetings and other promotional media. Ideas for program materials include:

- Video presentations with follow-up discussion
- Talks by outside experts, such as fire and police department representatives
- Contests that create awareness and interest
- Testimonials by employees who were injured or who escaped injury through good safety practices

☐ Conclusion

Safety motivational programs improve safety performance on the job as well as off the job by working in concert with the facility's fundamental safety program. There are two principal types of motivational programs: promotional programs, which deliver messages that make safety visible to employees and lead to increased safety awareness; and incentive programs, which motivate employees to work safely by rewarding and recognizing individual and group contributions to safety. For these programs to be effective, they must be managed in the same manner as other business programs, working toward achieving goals and delineating responsibilities.

Table 15-2. The Top 10 Employee Off-the-Job Disabling-Injury Categories of 1993, Four Major Manufacturers

Home	Public	Transportation
Cuts on sharp objects	Falls, slips	Automobile, truck, recreational vehicle
Falls, slips	Fights, assaults	Motorcycle, moped
Lifting, pushing, pulling (sprains/strains)	Lifting, pushing, pulling (sprains/strains)	
Struck by falling or flying objects	Sports (outdoors/indoors)	

Source: *Off-the-Job Safety Program Manual.* Chicago: National Safety Council, 1993.

Table 15-3. Program Topics, by Season

	Traffic	Home	Public
Spring	New signs, signals, pavement markings Motorcycles Recreational vehicles Vehicle maintenance Vacation safety	Poison Prevention Week—third week in March Spring cleanup, fixup	Bike safety/helmets Boat inspection and maintenance Personal flotation devices
Summer	Trailer—towing Hot-weather vehicle maintenance—cooling, system, tires	Lawn mowers and other powered garden equipment Backyard pools Pesticides and insecticides—how to choose and use them Lifting-lowering, pushing-pulling injuries	Safe Boating Week—first week in June Safe swimming Sun hazards—sunburn, sunstroke, heat exhaustion Fishing safety Camping safety Racket sports—tennis, racquetball, squash
Fall	Back to school—young pedestrians Winter car maintenance—battery, snow tires, chains, defroster check	Fire Prevention Week—week including Oct. 9 (in remembrance of Chicago Fire, Oct. 9, 1871) Halloween Safety Home heating-system checkup	Contact sports—personal protective equipment Hunting safety Farm Safety Week—third week in September
Winter	How to "jump start" a car Winter driving techniques—how to avoid getting stuck, how to handle a skid, etc. Snowmobiles in traffic	Holiday safety—"Send them home sober" Toy selection Outdoor falls due to ice and snow Snow thrower safety and heart attack warnings for shovelers	Winter sports—hockey, ice skating, skiing, tobogganing and sledding, snowmobiling Frostbite and hypothermia
Year-Round	Railroad grade crossings Defensive driving Occupant protection—safety belts, child restraints Alcohol and other drug abuse Two-wheelers—bicycles, mopeds, minibikes Roadside hazards	Slips and falls Care and use of hand and power tools Home fire safety—exit drills, smoke detectors, sprinklers	Sports—physical conditioning First aid Cardiopulmonary resuscitation Eye protection

Source: *Off-the-Job Safety Program Manual.* Chicago: National Safety Council, 1993.

Safety Program Evaluation

Once safety and health program elements are in place, an ongoing process of evaluation must be carried out. Its purpose is to measure the achievement of established goals and to evaluate program outcomes, such as trend analysis and program effectiveness. These evaluations also are necessary to meet OSHA and JCAHO requirements for an annual review of the facility's overall safety program effectiveness.

This chapter describes the steps involved in developing an ongoing evaluation process for the facility's safety program. It also discusses annual evaluations and the use of safety program evaluation as a tool for resource allocation.

□ Ongoing Program Evaluation

Developing an evaluation process basically involves five steps. These are:

1. Identify program elements
2. Select specific indicators
3. Develop a sampling plan
4. Collect the data
5. Analyze the data

Step 1. Identify Program Elements

The first step in developing the evaluation process is to identify all the safety and health elements that must be monitored. These include:

- Program administration
- Information management
- Patient safety
- Education and training
- Hazardous materials
- Bloodborne pathogens
- Emergency preparedness
- Fire safety
- Incident reporting and investigation
- Safety motivation

Step 2. Select Specific Indicators

The second step of the process is to select specific indicators that will measure the effectiveness of each element and signal when corrective action needs to be taken. Usually, three indicators will provide a basis for evaluation; however, additional indicators may be needed depending on program type and how well it is working. The elements and typical indicators are:

- Policies and procedures
  - Are policies and procedures in place?
  - Are they current?
  - Do observations show that employees are following the procedures?
- Training
  - Do records show that all employees are trained?
  - Do employees demonstrate that they know the procedures through either written or verbal testing?
  - Is a process in place to retrain employees who do not know the procedures?
- Ongoing monitoring and corrective action
  - Is a process in place to monitor the performance of all programs?
  - Have indicators and monitoring frequencies been established based on sound statistical procedures?
  - Is there documentation and a tracking system of corrective action elements, responsibility, and timing for identified safety problems?

Step 3. Develop a Sampling Plan

The third step is to develop a sampling plan that specifies how much information must be collected and how it will be collected. Because this process requires data management skills, it is important that the individual responsible for establishing the program be trained in the statistical techniques of data collection. In addition, he or she must be trained in the use of computerized data management and analysis. Sound statistical data analysis will allow the facility to respond to safety problems and take corrective action to bring about change in safety performance, thereby avoiding reacting to data that are not statistically significant. Further, using a statistical approach will identify those elements of the safety program that can be measured and those that cannot. Many indicators provide insufficient data to allow statistical analysis over a short time span. In these cases, common sense and experience may be more effective in determining if corrective action is necessary.

Step 4. Collect the Data

The fourth step in the evaluation process is to actually collect the data based on information developed in the first three steps. Data can be collected using employee interviews and testing. Unannounced walk-through inspections by safety personnel and safety committee members also can be effective in uncovering equipment hazards and unsafe practices. Employees should be asked about their reactions to the practicality and effectiveness of various program elements. Additionally, department managers and supervisors can monitor daily practices. When employees are not working safely, managers should determine why, assuring employees that they want to know if the problem is one of poorly designed procedures or insufficient training. Managers and supervisors can explain that employee input is valuable to the sustained success of the safety program. This communication is essential, because line employees are the ones most responsible for daily implementation of the program. Another way to assess employee reactions to procedures is through the use of employee response to questions on in-service evaluation forms. Finally, in addition to discussions with employees, program effectiveness can be evaluated by observing departmental and facilitywide trends in incidents, injuries, and illnesses.

Step 5. Analyze the Data

The final step in program evaluation is to analyze the data in order to identify specific problems and trends requiring corrective action. The results of the analysis are then publicized to those organizations responsible for taking corrective action. In addition, the information is summarized and given to the safety committee for its use in overseeing and managing the overall safety program. Summaries of the indicators and corrective actions taken are compiled and issued by the safety committee in minutes and quarterly reports.

☐ Annual Program Evaluation

In addition to ongoing program evaluation, the facility must evaluate the overall safety program on an annual basis. This evaluation is developed as a report that usually is issued by the safety committee. The report shows progress and accomplishments using monitoring data and information from all the committee and subcommittee reports. It should spell out what the previous goals were and if they were met. It also should specify the goals for the coming year.

A number of other sources of information may be used to prepare the report. These include:

- Incident, illness, and injury reports
- Voluntary and regulatory agency survey reports
- Insurance company inspection results
- Workers' compensation statistics
- New and old policies and procedures

All elements of the safety and health program should be covered in the annual report. The report is vital because it (1) provides a well-documented analysis of the effectiveness of the total safety management program and (2) specifies the facility's performance improvement strategy.

☐ Evaluation of New and Revised Safety Programs

Although ongoing evaluation is adequate for programs that are proven to be effective, a more complete evaluation of new or revised programs should be undertaken six months after implementation. The purpose of this evaluation is to ensure that new procedures have been fully implemented, that they are accomplishing what they were designed to accomplish, and that they are achieving this in an acceptable manner. If the program has been revised as a result of a needs assessment, the review should utilize the results of the original needs assessment as a basis for determining progress.

Even though the first evaluation should take place approximately six months after implementation of a new program element, dramatic results should not be expected immediately. Developing and implementing the policies and procedures, introducing them to staff, and training employees in carrying them out may require reevaluation and development of new performance goals.

Without the tools of evaluation and consistent monitoring, any program could suffer after the initial push for implementation. Ongoing review and measurement of results is essential in determining what the program has accomplished and where future effort should be focused.

☐ Program Evaluation as a Tool for Resource Allocation

Most facilities face an ongoing problem of managing safety in regards to the demands on certain resources. These include:

- Cost reduction
- Rapid facility growth
- Increased government regulation

Frequently, safety resources, both manpower and financial, are cut because of the lack of measurable accomplishments. In addition, often the consequences of meeting safety regulatory requirements are not adequately communicated to upper management.

Facility growth causes major changes in services or other processes that make some policies and procedures obsolete, and necessitate major revisions in existing procedures. For example, as the demographics of society change, facilities may move toward expanded services for the elderly, whose needs differ from those of younger patients. In addition, facility growth means the use of equipment relying on advanced technology, requiring stepped-up training for users, stricter safety monitoring, and preventive maintenance.

Government and other regulations are changing at a steady pace and require alteration in practices that once were routine. Stricter enforcement and penalties make adherence to new standards even more important, because fines can affect the facility's earnings. Many regulations are complex and require significant resources to implement and maintain compliance.

Because of these assaults on resources, safety program management must keep pace by using the best safety management technology and processes available. An important benefit of program evaluation is that it can define the most effective use of available resources. The knowledge gained through evaluation enables the safety committee to prioritize resource allocation to programs that are not meeting goals. In addition, where there are insufficient resources allocated to correct existing program deficiencies and implement new programs, information from the evaluation process will provide the data to support the need for additional resources. One of the responsibilities of the safety committee is to ensure that the chief executive officer, board, administrators, and others involved in resource allocation are aware of the consequences of cutting back on specific program support.

☐ Conclusion

An evaluation process is essential to ensure the continued success of the facility's safety program. Ongoing evaluation involves selection of the safety elements that need to be evaluated and use of statistically based indicators to provide the data for the evaluation. In addition, the facility must develop a written annual report summarizing the information from the ongoing evaluation process. The annual reports inform administration of the safety program's needs, progress, and accomplishments.

List of Organizations

American Conference of Governmental Industrial Hygienists
1330 Kemper Meadow Drive
Cincinnati, OH 45240
513/742-2020

American Health Care Association
1201 L Street, N.W.
Washington, DC 20005
202/842-4444

American Hospital Association
One North Franklin
Chicago, IL 60606
312/422-3000

American Industrial Hygiene Association
2700 Prosperity Avenue, Suite 250
Fairfax, VA 22031-4307
703/849-8888

American National Standards Institute
11 West 42nd Street, Thirteenth Floor
New York, NY 10036
212/642-4900

American Society of Safety Engineers
1800 East Oakton Street
Des Plaines, IL 60018-2187
708/692-4121

American Society for Training and Development
1640 King Street, Box 1443
Alexandria, VA 22313-2043
703/683-8100

Association of Air Medical Services
35 South Raymond Avenue, Suite 205
Pasadena, CA 91105-1931
818/793-1232

Centers for Disease Control and Prevention
1600 Clifton Road, N.E.
Atlanta, GA 30333
404/639-3534

Compressed Gas Association
1725 Jefferson Davis Highway, Suite 1004
Arlington, VA 22202-4102
703/412-0900

Department of Transportation
400 7th Street, S.W.
Washington, DC 20590
202/366-4000

Federal Aviation Administration
800 Independence Avenue, S.W.
Washington, DC 20591
202/267-3883

Federal Emergency Management Agency
500 C Street, S.W.
Washington, DC 20472
202/646-4600

Federal Register
Superintendent of Documents
U.S. Government Printing Office
Washington, DC 20402
202/783-3238

Golden Shoe Club
Hy-Test, Inc.
312 Wilson Drive
Jefferson City, MO 65109
800/633-4987

Joint Commission on Accreditation of Healthcare Organizations
One Renaissance Boulevard
Oakbrook Terrace, IL 60181
708/916-5600

Mine Safety and Health Administration
Department of Labor
4015 Wilson Boulevard
Arlington, VA 22203
703/235-1452

Office of Emergency Preparedness—National Disaster Medical System
U.S. Department of Health and Human Services
5600 Fishers Lane
Parklawn Building, Room 4-81
Rockville, MD 20857
301/443-1167

National Fire Protection Association
One Batterymarch Park
Quincy, MA 02269
617/770-3000

National Institute for Occupational Safety and Health
Hubert H. Humphrey Building
200 Independence Avenue, S.W., Room 715H
Washington, DC 20201
202/690-7134

National Restaurant Association
1200 17th Street, N.W.
Washington, DC 20036
202/331-5900

National Safety Council
1121 Spring Lake Drive
Itasca, IL 60143-3201
708/285-1121

National Weather Service
Commerce Department
National Oceanic and Atmospheric Administration
1325 East-West Highway
Silver Spring, MD 20910
301/713-0689

Nuclear Regulatory Commission
Washington, DC 20555
301/492-7000

Occupational Safety and Health Administration
200 Constitution Avenue
Washington, DC 20210
202/219-7031

Orange County Emergency Medical Services Agency
517 North Main Street, Room 301
Santa Ana, CA 92701
714/568-4283

Prevent Blindness America
500 East Remington Road
Schaumburg, IL 60173
708/843-2020

State of California Emergency Medical Services Authority
1930 Ninth Street, Suite 100
Sacramento, CA 95814
916/322-4336

Underwriters Laboratories
333 Pfingsten Road
Northbrook, IL 60062
708/272-8800

U.S. Environmental Protection Agency
Office of Solid Waste and Emergency Response
401 M Street, S.W.
Washington, DC 20460
202/260-2090

U.S. Food and Drug Administration
900 Madison Avenue
Baltimore, MD 21201
410/962-3396

U.S. Practitioner Reporting Network
United States Pharmacopeia
12601 Twinbrook Parkway
Rockville, MD 20852
800/638-6725

Glossary of Abbreviations

ADA	Americans with Disabilities Act
AHA	American Hospital Association
AIDS	Acquired Immunodeficiency Syndrome
ANSI	American National Standards Institute
ASHBEAMS	American Society of Hospital-Based Emergency Air Medical Services
BBPS	Bloodborne Pathogens Standard
CAA	Clean Air Act of 1970
CDC	Centers for Disease Control and Prevention
CDT	Cumulative Trauma Disorders
CEPP	Chemical Emergency Preparedness Program (EPA)
CERCLA	Comprehensive Environmental Response Compensation Liability Act
CFR	Code of Federal Regulations
CGA	Compressed Gas Association
CSHO	Compliance Safety and Health Officer
CWA	Clean Water Act of 1977
DOL	Department of Labor
DOT	Department of Transportation
ECT	Electroconvulsive Therapy
EMS	Emergency Medical Services
EPA	U.S. Environmental Protection Agency
FAA	Federal Aviation Authority
FDA	Food and Drug Administration
FEMA	Federal Emergency Management Agency
HBV	Hepatitis B Virus
HHS	Department of Health and Human Services
HIV	Human Immunodeficiency Virus
ILSM	Interim Life Safety Measures
JCAHO	Joint Commission on Accreditation of Healthcare Organizations (Joint Commission)
LASER	Light Amplification by Stimulated Emission of Radiation
MSDS	Material Safety Data Sheet
NFPA	National Fire Protection Association
NIOSH	National Institute for Occupational Safety and Health
NPDES	National Pollutant Discharge Elimination System
NRC	Nuclear Regulatory Commission
NSC	National Safety Council
NTP	National Toxicology Program

OES	Office of Emergency Services
OSHA	Occupational Safety and Health Administration
PICE	Potential Injury Creating Event
PPE	Personal Protective Equipment
RCRA	Resource Conservation and Recovery Act
RQ	Reportable Quantity
SARA	Superfund Amendments and Reauthorization Act of 1986
SIC	Standard Industrial Code
SMDA	Safe Medical Device Act
TB	Tuberculosis
TPQ	Threshold Planning Quantity
TSCA	Toxic Substances Control Act of 1976

Hazard Surveillance Checklist

The following checklist covers many topics for consideration during hazard surveillance visual inspections. Because the functions and structure of each facility vary, it may be necessary to add questions addressing the particular needs of individual facilities. The items are numbered by group to allow the addition of other questions without causing numbering conflicts. The first group of items addresses facilitywide safety concerns. Following groups address concerns particular to certain departments. Items from the facilitywide category have been repeated in some departmental categories in which the items are especially important.

The individual responsible for a visual inspection should note hazards on the Hazard Surveillance Reporting Log located at the end of the checklist. This log provides a formal means of problem documentation, recommended action, and action taken. After the visual inspection is complete, the Hazard Surveillance Reporting Log is submitted to the safety committee for analysis and action on the safety problems that require committee action.

Item		Yes	No
	Facilitywide		
1-1	Does electrical equipment have grounded connections (three-pronged plugs)?		
1-2	Are electrical cords in good condition?		
1-3	Is adequate ventilation provided in areas where hazardous materials are being used?		
1-4	Are unused materials, equipment, and supplies stored away?		
1-5	Is storage arranged to allow adequate work space, ease of access, and room for employees to bend their knees for a proper lifting technique?		
1-6	Are cabinets provided in each department for small tools, buckets, brooms, mops, etc.?		
1-7	Are all items being stored off the floor?		
1-8	Is storage on ledges, cabinet tops, radiators, tops of lockers, etc., eliminated?		
1-9	Are fire alarm pull boxes easily accessible?		
1-10	Are evacuation routes posted in each area?		
1-11	Are fire extinguishers easily accessible?		
1-12	Are fire extinguishers charged?		
1-13	Is all storage at least 18 inches below sprinkler heads?		
1-14	Are fire doors, aisles, and exits clear?		

Item		Yes	No
1-15	Are all exit signs illuminated?		
1-16	Do all exit doors swing outward?		
1-17	Do exit doors have working panic hardware or fire exit hardware?		
1-18	Do exit doors unlock from the inside?		
1-19	Are switches on heavy equipment recessed or otherwise guarded?		
1-20	Are switches located so that employees do not have to lean on or against metal equipment to reach them?		
1-21	Are switches on heavy equipment located so as to enable rapid emergency cutoff?		
1-22	Are guards provided to prevent injury from electrical shock, rotating blades, etc.?		
1-23	Are portable ladders unpainted and sturdy with nonslip bases? If freestanding, do they have a metal spreader or locking device?		
1-24	Are fixed ladders securely anchored?		
1-25	Are broken ladders destroyed or tagged and removed from service?		
1-26	Do stairs and ramps have handrails?		
1-27	Are stairway treads in good condition?		
1-28	Are stairway riser height and tread width uniform?		
1-29	Are No Smoking restrictions observed?		
1-30	Are cleaning solutions or other hazardous chemicals stored in closed containers?		
1-31	Are material safety data sheets readily available?		
1-32	Are mops available for cleaning up spills?		
1-33	Do employees remove protruding nails, metal strapping, and wires from containers before handling?		
1-34	Is protective clothing and equipment provided in all areas where employees are exposed to hazards including dangerous chemicals, vapors, and noise?		
1-35	Are all employees wearing sturdy, closed-toe, low-heeled shoes?		
1-36	Do employees moving heavy materials wear steel-toed shoes or strap-on metal foot shields?		
	Materials Management		
2-1	Are operating instructions posted near sterilization units?		
2-2	Is the area clear of broken glass?		
2-3	Is nonskid flooring provided near decontamination equipment where floors are often wet?		
2-4	Are there color contrasts on the edges of loading docks and ramps?		
2-5	Are storage shelves sturdy?		
2-6	Are battery-charging areas well ventilated?		
	Housekeeping		
3-1	Are all lighting fixtures functioning?		
3-2	Is a sign posted to warn individuals of wet areas?		

Item		Yes	No
3-3	Are nonskid waxes or polishes used?		
3-4	If lightweight rugs are used, do they have rubber backing?		
3-5	Are the proper tools available for opening containers?		
3-6	Are flammable liquids stored in closed containers?		
3-7	Are cabinets containing flammables clearly labeled?		
3-8	Are plastic liners in all garbage pails?		
3-9	Are all garbage pails covered?		
3-10	Are there special receptacles for disposal of needles and other sharp objects?		
3-11	Are trash cans in patient rooms free of nonpaper waste?		
3-12	Are cleaning solutions clearly labeled with ingredients and warnings indicated?		

Laundry

4-1	Are eye and hand protective equipment provided for employees handling cleaning solutions?		
4-2	Are steam lines insulated to prevent burns?		
4-3	Is the safety on the feed roll of the flat ironer in working order?		
4-4	Are special bags and markers available for contagious linen?		
4-5	Are employees who sort contagious linen protected with gowns, masks, and gloves?		
4-6	Are floors clear of standing water, grease, etc.?		
4-7	Are dryers free of lint?		
4-8	Is equipment free of excess oil and grease?		
4-9	Are mats or nonskid flooring provided in wet areas?		
4-10	Are employees wearing nonskid shoes?		
4-11	Are portable air fans guarded?		
4-12	Is hot equipment shielded to protect employees from the heat?		
4-13	Do employees have easy access to water and cool air to combat heat stress?		
4-14	Is disinfectant soap available in the laundry?		
4-15	Are carts clearly designated for dirty or clean laundry?		
4-16	Are instructions for proper operation of laundry equipment posted?		

Maintenance and Engineering

5-1	Are oily rags kept in closed metal containers?		
5-2	Are all hand tools stored in their proper places when not in use?		
5-3	Are wrench jaws in good condition so that they will not slip?		
5-4	Are wrenches and sockets available in various sizes so that the proper size is available for each task?		
5-5	Are chisel, pin, and punch heads free of mushrooming?		
5-6	Are hammer heads unchipped, and are their handles tight and free of cracks?		
5-7	Do saws have blade guards?		

Item		Yes	No
5-8	Are tools out of patient reach?		
5-9	Are walkways in good repair and unobstructed?		
5-10	Are direction signs properly lighted, placed, and easy to read?		
5-11	Are guardrails and gratings in place to prevent individuals from falling into stairwells?		
5-12	Are nonmetal ladders available for working on electrical equipment and changing light bulbs?		
5-13	Is gasoline-powered equipment used in well-ventilated areas?		
5-14	Are oxygen cylinders stored away from combustibles, especially oil and grease.		
5-15	Are stored oxygen cylinders separated from fuel gas cylinders by at least 20 feet?		
5-16	Are full and empty gas cylinders stored separately?		
5-17	Are all compressed gas cylinders chained or otherwise secured?		
5-18	Are all cylinders stored away from heat sources such as radiators, steam pipes, and direct sunlight?		
5-19	Are trash compactors operable only in the closed position?		
5-20	Are there safety measures or devices on trash compactors (such as two-hand controls, electric eyes, or emergency shut-off bars) to minimize risk of injury?		
5-21	Is there adequate ventilation in areas where paint is used?		

Business Offices

Item		Yes	No
6-1	Are file cabinets anchored?		
6-2	Are wrist rests, glare screens, and footrests available?		
6-3	Are current safety and disaster manuals available?		

Operating Room

Item		Yes	No
7-1	Are wall plates for doors operational?		
7-2	Are humidity and temperature gauges operational?		
7-3	Are restricted access signs in place?		
7-4	Are compressed gas tanks secured?		
7-5	Are laser and X-ray warning lights operational?		
7-6	Are containers for the discard of sharp objects available?		
7-7	Are chemicals labeled?		
7-8	Are medical gas lines labeled?		
7-9	Is the emergency call system operational?		

Laboratory

Item		Yes	No
8-1	Are chemical and biological safety hoods operational?		
8-2	Is the emergency eye wash and shower operational?		
8-3	Are spill kits provided?		
8-4	Are chemicals labeled?		

Item		Yes	No
	Emergency Department		
9-1	Is the emergency call system operational?		
9-2	Are compressed gas cylinders secured?		
9-3	Are emergency power circuits operational?		
9-4	Are controlled drugs secured when not it use?		
	Radiology and Nuclear Medicine		
10-1	Are chemicals labeled?		
10-2	Are chemical and radiation spill kits available?		
10-3	Are hot labs separated from the rest of the department?		
10-4	Is ventilation provided in developing and processing areas?		
	Nursing		
11-1	Do all beds have side rails?		
11-2	Are side rails raised at night for all patients?		
11-3	Are wheelchair locks engaged when stationary?		
11-4	Are seat belts present on wheelchairs?		
11-5	Are footrests on wheelchairs in working order?		
11-6	Are call buttons within easy reach of patients?		
11-7	Are designated receptacles available for broken syringes, needles, and empty bottles wherever medications and treatments are given?		
11-8	Do employees use proper methods for lifting patients?		
11-9	Is wiring adequate in all areas to avoid routine use of extension cords?		
11-10	Are floors free from breaks, loose tiles or linoleum, or any obstruction that might cause people to stumble or fall?		
11-11	Are handles provided on all mattresses?		
11-12	Are medicine cabinets and carts locked when not in use?		
11-13	Are gas cylinders chained or otherwise secured to the carrier?		
11-14	Are gas cylinders chained while in storage?		
11-15	Are gas cylinders secured when empty?		
11-16	Is a valve protection cap in place on oxygen cylinders not in use?		
11-17	Are No Smoking signs posted on oxygen tents?		
11-18	Are electrical cords placed so as to prevent tripping hazards?		
11-19	Are acids and other chemicals properly labeled and stored?		
	Physical Therapy		
12-1	Are floors made of or covered with nonslip material where instructions are given for walking with crutches, canes, and walkers?		
12-2	Is equipment available for testing oil, water, and paraffin temperatures?		
12-3	Are mops available in areas where baths are given?		

Item		Yes	No
12-4	Are ropes, pulleys, straps, etc., in good condition?		
12-5	Are wall or ceiling brackets firmly attached?		
	Storerooms		
13-1	Are storerooms well lit?		
13-2	Are storerooms clear of empty cartons and other rubbish?		
13-3	Are heavy items stored on lower shelves?		
13-4	Are liquids stored below eye level?		
13-5	Are portable and stationary storage racks in safe condition (free from broken or bent shelves and set on solid legs)?		
13-6	Are objects that might roll blocked?		
13-7	Are cases or boxes crisscrossed when stacked higher than six feet?		
13-8	Are storage shelves adequate for the weight involved?		
13-9	Are corrugated cartons opened with a sharp knife or other appropriate tool?		
	Food Services		
14-1	Is a routine inspection for breakage and spill hazards made after each meal?		
14-2	Has faulty or damaged equipment been removed from use?		
14-3	Are there restrictions or guidelines on loose-fitting clothing, jewelry, and long hair to prevent entanglement in machinery, contamination of food, and fire while near range burners?		
14-4	Are push sticks used to feed food grinders and choppers?		
14-5	Are storage facilities sufficient to provide shelf or rack space for all supplies, eliminating temporary storage on counter or table surfaces?		
14-6	Is china stored in short stacks?		
14-7	Are cups and glassware stored rim edge down?		
14-8	Do employees carry only small stacks of glassware?		
14-9	Are all glassware and china free of cracks and chips?		
14-10	Are broken glassware and china placed in a marked receptacle from which they can be dumped, not handpicked?		
14-11	Are tops removed from glass bottles before discarding them to avoid explosion if accidentally burned?		
14-12	Is ice chipping done in nonglass containers?		
14-13	Is glassware kept on separate racks from silver and china?		
14-14	Is equipment for opening crates, barrels, and cartons (hammer, wire cutter, pliers, and cardboard carton openers) provided?		
14-15	Are handtrucks available for moving bulk supplies?		
14-16	Are crates and cartons opened away from open food containers?		
14-17	Are garbage cans leak-proof?		
14-18	Do cupboards have sliding doors or are swinging doors kept closed?		

Item		Yes	No
14-19	Is storage of foodstuffs separate from storage of cleaning supplies and other poisonous substances?		
14-20	Is the refrigerator located so that its door does not swing into and block a major traffic way or corridor when opened?		
14-21	Are nonbreakable containers used where possible?		
14-22	Are flame- and oven-proof glass and ceramic containers allowed to warm between removal from refrigeration and use in an oven or on a stove?		
14-23	Is a device installed to permit exit from the inside of walk-in refrigerators?		
14-24	Are screen or mesh guards provided around blower fans in walk-in refrigerators?		
14-25	Are crevices and trays on ranges free of grease?		
14-26	Are utensil handles turned away from burners, pilot lights, and the front of the stove?		
14-27	Are pot holders in good condition?		
14-28	Do employees use only dry pot holders?		
14-29	To view a cooking item, do employees lift the side of the lid away from them to prevent steam burns?		
14-30	Do employees stand to one side to light a gas oven and check for ignition before closing the oven door?		
14-31	Are grease drippings removed from the broiler after each use?		
14-32	When carrying food to the dining room, do employees load trays with the heaviest items in the center?		
14-33	Is the traffic flow orderly so that attendants do not collide?		
14-34	Is there a window in the door between the serving area and the dining room?		
14-35	Is each side of swinging doors marked In or Out?		
14-36	If necessary, are doors between the serving area and the dining area prevented from swinging into a traffic area by a rail that restricts door opening to 90 degrees and prevents individuals from walking into the door?		
14-37	Is traffic-free storage space provided for carts used to transport food?		
14-38	Is food transported to patient rooms by cart whenever possible?		
14-39	Are tables available in patient rooms on which to place food trays?		
14-40	Are dish racks kept off the floor to prevent tripping hazards?		
14-41	Are drain boards large enough for draining without pyramid stacking?		
14-42	Do employees drain sinks before removing broken china and glass?		
14-43	Do sinks permit draining without employees having to reach into the water?		
14-44	Are rubber gloves provided for dishwashers?		
14-45	Do employees use correct amounts of detergents and other cleaning agents?		
14-46	Is a thermometer used to test water temperature before washing dishes?		
14-47	Are dishes and glasses washed separately from pots?		
14-48	Are knives sharp and in good condition?		
14-49	Are cuts always made away from the body?		
14-50	Are blades stored with the cutting edge covered?		
14-51	Are heavy lids on equipment such as steam kettles secured to prevent accidental falling?		

Hazard Reporting Log

Reported by: _____   Survey Date: _____

Date Reported	Comments/Action Recommended	Action Taken	Date Resolved

Bibliography

Baxter Ergonomics Guidelines. Deerfield, IL: Baxter, 1993.

Behling, D., and Guy, J. Hazards of the healthcare profession. *Occupational Health and Safety* 62(2):54-57, Feb. 1993.

Chaff & Co. *Building a Successful Safety Committee.* Signal Mountain, TN: Chaff & Co., 1992.

ECRI. Cellular phones could pose patient risks. *Health Technology Trends* 5(9):2, Sept. 1993.

Feuerstein, P. Incentives inspire safe behavior. *Safety and Health* 145(1):42-45, Jan. 1992.

Glasson, L. The care of psychiatric patients in the emergency department. *Journal of Emergency Nursing* 19(5):385-91, Oct. 1993.

Glasson, L. Change in the health care field: confronting the issues. *Journal of Healthcare Protection Management* 9(2):40-43, Summer 1993.

Henry, V. H. Make sure you know your legal rights when OSHA arrives at your facility. *Industrial Fire World* 7(2):9-14, Mar.-Apr. 1992, and 7(3):9-14, May-June 1992.

Hislop, R. D. Developing a safety incentive program. *Professional Safety* 31(4):20-25, Apr. 1993.

Janowiak, J. Incentive programs: only the icing, not the cake. *Safety and Health* 148(1):62-65, July 1993.

Joint Commission on Accreditation of Healthcare Organizations. Documentation of fire drills simplified in AMH. *Joint Commission Perspectives* 3(2):7, Mar.-Apr. 1993.

Joint Commission on Accreditation of Healthcare Organizations. *The Measurement Mandate.* Oakbrook Terrace, IL: JCAHO, 1993.

Key, M. J. *How to Start and Promote a Safety Award Program.* St. Paul, MN: Five Star Publishing, 1987.

Lathrop, J. K., editor. *Life Safety Code Handbook, Fifth Edition.* Quincy, MA: National Fire Protection Association, 1991.

McLarney, V. J., and Chaff, L. F., editors. *Effective Health Care Facilities Management.* Chicago: American Hospital Publishing, 1991.

National Safety Council. *1993 Accident Facts.* Itasca, IL: NSC, 1993.

National Safety Council. *Supervisors' Safety Manual, 7th Edition.* Chicago: NSC, 1991.

Newman, M., and Kachuba, J. B. *Monitoring Chemical Exposures in Healthcare Institutions.* Cincinnati: Healthcare Environments Press, 1993.

Occupational Safety and Health Administration. *All About OSHA.* Washington, DC: OSHA, 1991.

Occupational Safety and Health Administration. *Framework for a Comprehensive Health and Safety Program in the Hospital Environment.* Washington, DC: OSHA, 1993.

Peterson, D. Establishing good "safety culture" helps mitigate workplace dangers. *Occupational Health and Safety* 62(7):20-24, July 1993.

Phoon, W. H., and Lee, H. S. Hearing protection plans require proper ear plug selection, usage. *Occupational Health and Safety* 62(5):98-117, May 1993.

Pritchett, P., and Pound, R. *High-Velocity Culture Change.* Dallas: Pritchett, 1993.

Revising your fire safety plans. *Hospital Security and Safety Management* 14(8):5, Dec. 1993.

Safety Management Services. *Continuous Improvement for Safety Training.* Mt. Prospect, IL: Safety Management Services, 1991.

Thurber, S. Teach your workers to take safe habits home. *Safety and Health* 147(6):62-66, June 1993.

U.S. Department of Health and Human Services. *Guidelines for Protecting the Safety and Health of Health Care Workers.* Washington, DC: DHHS, 1988.

U.S. Equal Employment Opportunity Commission. *A Technical Assistance Manual on the Employment Provisions (Title I) of the Americans with Disabilities Act.* Washington, DC: EEOC, 1992.

Index

(continued on next page)

Additional Books of Interest

High Technology in Health Care: Risk Management Perspectives

edited by Robin A. Maley, M.P.H., R.N., and Alice L. Epstein, M.H.A.

This book examines the risks associated with the acquisition and use of current high-technology equipment and suggests techniques to prevent or reduce those risks. Covers some of the legal and ethical issues surrounding various new and high-risk procedures and provides guidelines for actions to deter risks that compromise patient safety and the financial solvency of the institution.

Catalog No. E99-178158 (must be included when ordering)
1993. 296 pages.
$62.00 (AHA members, $49.00)

Managing Health Care Construction Projects: A Practical Guide

compiled by Michael Hemmes

A collection of practical, how-to articles collected from *Health Facilities Management* magazine that will provide assistance as you plan, manage, and control large and small construction projects. The book helps you decide between renovation and new construction, organize internal project teams, recruit outside project managers, and select architects.

Catalog No. E99-055100 (must be included when ordering)
1993. 156 pages, 23 figures.
$42.50 (AHA members, $32.50)

Managing Hospital Materials Management

by Kowalski-Dickow Associates, Inc., in cooperation with the American Society for Healthcare Materials Management of the AHA

A comprehensive treatment of the core functions of materials management principles and practices. Illustrates to other managers how materials management concepts and methods can be applied to their department.

Catalog No. E99-142101 (must be included when ordering)
1993. 332 pages, 99 figures, 47 tables.
$65.00 (AHA members, $52.00)

To order, call TOLL FREE
1-800-AHA-2626